THE UNFRAGILE MIND

THE
UNFRAGILE MIND

MAKING SENSE OF MENTAL HEALTH

GAVIN FRANCIS

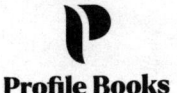
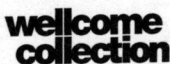

First published in Great Britain in 2026 by
Profile Books Ltd
29 Cloth Fair
London
EC1A 7JQ
www.profilebooks.co.uk

Published in association with Wellcome Collection

**wellcome
collection**

183 Euston Road
London NW1 2BE
www.wellcomecollection.org

Typeset in Dante by MacGuru Ltd
Printed and bound in Great Britain by
CPI Group (UK) Ltd, Croydon CR0 4YY

A CIP catalogue record for this book is available from the British Library.

Our product safety representative in the EU is BGC Sustainability & Compliance, 7 avenue du Général Leclerc, Paris, 75014, France
https://baldwinglobalconsulting.com

ISBN 978 1 80081 975 7
eISBN 978 1 80081 976 4
Audio 978 1 80522 888 2

wellcome collection

for my patients,
in gratitude for their trust,

& also

for Andrew Franklin:
publisher, editor and friend

The majority of people who have psychological problems are seen and treated by their general practitioner, and only a small proportion are referred to hospital psychiatrists.

R. I. Cohen and J. J. Hart, *An Introduction to Psychiatry*

Our normal waking consciousness, rational consciousness as we call it, is but one special type of consciousness, whilst all about it, parted from it by the filmiest of screens, there lie potential forms of consciousness entirely different.

William James, *The Varieties of Religious Experience*

We all build internal sea walls to keep at bay the sadnesses of life and the often overwhelming forces within our minds. In whatever way we do this – through love, work, family, faith, friends, denial, alcohol, drugs, or medication – we build these walls, stone by stone, over a lifetime.

Kay Redfield Jamison, *An Unquiet Mind*

CONTENTS

Just as physicians must honour the privileged access they have to our minds and our bodies, so they must honour the trust with which we share our stories. Even as long as 2,500 years ago that obligation was recognised: the Hippocratic Oath insists, 'Whatsoever in the course of practice you see or hear that ought never to be published abroad, you will not divulge.' As a doctor who is also a writer I've spent a great deal of time deliberating over that use of 'ought', considering what can and cannot be said without betraying the confidence of my patients.

The reflections that follow are grounded in my clinical experience, but the patients in them have been so disguised as to be unrecognisable – any similarities that remain are coincidental. Protecting confidences is an essential part of what I do: 'confidence' means 'with faith' – we are all patients sooner or later; we all want faith that we'll be heard, and that our privacy will be respected.

ADVENTURES IN THINKING, FEELING & BEING

You doctors come across so many odd people and are mixed up in so many strange situations. You know more of real life than anybody else, I am sure you have a lot to tell us if you want to.

Axel Munthe, *The Story of San Michele*

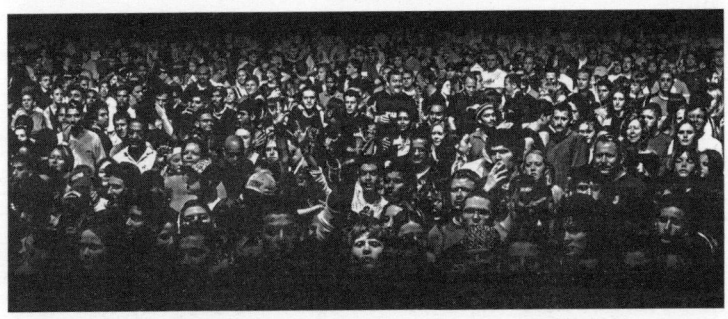

Look at the faces in a crowd: each one conceals a unique and intimate human drama. Every life is difficult sometimes, and to practise medicine is to be given the uncommon privilege of seeing through the facades we hide behind.

This is a book about states of mind and how we make sense of them. Most categories of mental health and illness are controversial because they are subjective: evolved over centuries through conversations between doctors and patients,

patients and patients and doctors and doctors, rather than arrived at through objective scientific tests. 'Patient' means 'sufferer', and suffering comes to us all.

The life of the mind is social; human relationships are as important to it as the function of brain cells. When a mind goes awry it does so in ways made available by the culture that formed it, and the one that surrounds it. The size and structure of the human brain haven't changed much in the last 300,000 years, but approaches to mental health and illness change all the time. A century from now our current approaches to psychology and psychiatry will seem at best quaint, at worst barbaric. But as the science of the mind expands, and more is understood, it's certain that kindness and compassion will remain central to good mental health care. Doctors study disease, but 'ease' should be their goal – the relief of human suffering, whether it be of body or mind.

Some of the best doctors I've known have also been the most humble, able to acknowledge the limits of their understanding and capable of changing their views as new developments demand fresh explanations. There's no such thing as a final theory; pretending to certainty leads to a brittle rigidity when there is nothing in nature that doesn't flow, evolve, bend, spin and change. Our minds are not brittle or rigid, they are dynamic, resilient and adaptive: they are not fragile, but *un*fragile. Their capacity for change is part of their very nature.

In the course of my work I meet people whose lives feel blighted by feelings of anxiety and fear, who are depressed or manic, who have been traumatised or abused, who are psychotic or addicted. It's work that obliges me every day to ask questions about the nature of consciousness, of mood, and the elements that go into making a meaningful life.

This book sets out with a particular premise: that there are landscapes of the mind, and to practise medicine, journeying with the stories of others, is to be a kind of adventurer through its many realms. There are many ways of thinking, feeling and being, and doctors explore them through conversations in the consultation room. The word 'doctor' means 'teacher' or 'guide': sometimes I guide my patients through those landscapes well known to me; at other times it's my patients who guide me. Among the rewards of medical practice are seeing the ways people meet, transcend and accommodate the difficulties in their lives.

PART I

MAPS OF THE MIND

1

THE BOX OF DELIGHTS

There is a great deal of unmapped country within
us which would have to be taken into account in an
explanation of our gusts and storms.

George Eliot, *Daniel Deronda*

There are plenty of ways to injure your head as a kid: you
can fall from a rope swing onto packed earth; you can be
bouncing on a bed, jostled by a companion and smack your
temple on an unyielding piece of furniture; you can be learning how to do wheelies on your bike and fall over backwards
onto concrete; you can misjudge the robustness of a branch
and fall twenty feet from a tree. As a child I tried all of these
ways of braining myself and more, and each time had been
rewarded with a trip to the local hospital. By my teens I had
already seen inside my own skull a few times, through the
magic of X-rays.

Hospital was a place of clean white lines and sterilised
blue curtains, its air thick with the smell of antiseptic floor
cleaner. To be there was to feel cared for by confident, com-
petent people who, despite their brisk efficiency, seemed
possessed of great kindness. And on my brief, occasional
overnight stays I came to anticipate that same atmosphere
of care. I liked the rhythm of the nurses coming and going
between nightshift, morning and backshift; the daily offices

of the cleaners as they made their life-saving circuit of the wards; the porters, bustling and whistling, cracking jokes; the occasional, unpredictable arrival of the doctors themselves.

The scars on my scalp are testimony of those injuries, but so were the X-ray films the staff ordered, which in those days were printed on stiff acetate sheets, black as welding masks. Years later I returned to the same hospital as a qualified doctor and, searching the basement for notes on a patient who shared my surname, I came across my own file of X-rays: a buff cardboard wallet crammed with ghostly images of my childhood skull.

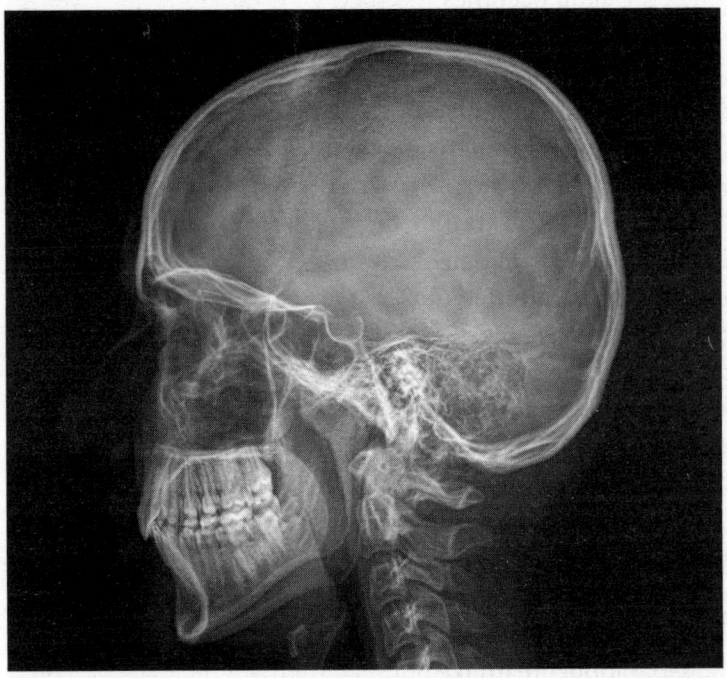

Even to a young child the skull is familiar from countless Halloween parodies; a universal symbol of mortality and the macabre. But when I held up images of my own skull to the buzzing strip lights there was only wonder: at the neat tangle of bone around the ears, the 'petrous' bone (hard as a rock, the same root as 'petrified'); the caverns of the sinuses above, behind and below the eyes, that change the resonance of the voice; the crisp rigidity of the jaw (the strongest bone of the body) with its row of socketed teeth; the little scoop of bone at the centre, round as a ladle, that saddles the pituitary gland – the body's hormonal headquarters. But what struck me most on seeing again my own childhood skull was the round think-bubble of the cranial 'vault', seemingly so empty because brain tissue doesn't show up on X-rays. In adults the skull becomes marbled with the imprint of veins – blood pumps over the brain so vigorously that its blood vessels thin the overlying bone. In a certain light the skull can be seen as the repository of all that makes us human, an ever-locked safe of the magical stuff of life.

In my teens I began to think of the brain in another way, as the origin and steersman of my mood. For years I was prone to episodes of plunging mood, a recurrent sinking feeling as if submerged in cold liquid, or perhaps encased by some invisible barrier that insulated me from all that felt good in the world, all that rendered life worth living. Sometimes the cloaking heaviness was still and cold, weighing on my sense of self like a leaden coat. At other times it was blurred, agitated and tremulous, and I'd feel stricken with fear over things undone, that may never be done, that may never happen, that I might never learn how to do.

I still catch faint echoes of that feeling of disconnection and separation, dreamlike but more like a nightmare, a heavy gut-ache of pervasive dread that has, mercifully, left me. In the bad years I'd drag myself from bed where I'd hardly slept, eat mechanically (choking back nausea), sit dazed on the bus in my barricaded world, ostensibly together with others though separated from them. It was a cold, dark place: I went through the motions of life, work and learning; in down times would walk in solitary loops, waiting for evening and home, while knowing that home brought no comfort. It was a nameless, shifting sense of unhappiness; I call it 'nameless' because my GP never felt it necessary to give it a name – a decision I now think was wise.

He was a man who'd known me since I could first walk. He recognised that I was lonely, and told me that the business of making friends is one of sharing: food, time, stories, secrets. He implied that my crash in mood was neither permanent nor inevitable, but was likely triggered by circumstance. It was a time of life beset by hormonal and social transitions, and my mind is one with a tendency to overthink. In the transformation from childhood into adolescence there had been a collapse in the relationships and activities that had kept me well.

And when, after a couple of years of misery, my mood began to lift, there was a buoyant sensation of relief and liberation, a rushing return of the ability to take pleasure in things, the return of the feeling of life and reward. Running, time and the fostering of new friendships were, in the end, what helped most. The friendships were difficult, because they required an ease with others that, in the beginning, it was necessary to fake.

The mind is pliable and suggestible, weaving its own reality from moment to moment, and it seems to me now that the lack of a formal diagnosis meant that I never felt locked into an expectation of feeling a certain way, or worried that my brain was in some way different from the brains of others, more sensitive or vulnerable to such lows. Denying it a label perhaps made it easier for me, when the time came, to shrug off that leaden coat.

If the opposite pole of depression is mania, the opposite

of anxiety might be inertia, a problem which occasionally finds its way into my office, manifesting as an inability to contemplate change. There are extreme versions of anxiety in which action becomes impossible – the idea of change itself becomes too frightening – but to be truly inert is to have no desire for change, and doesn't occasion the kind of abrasive, problematic behaviour that brings people into conflict with others the way psychosis or addiction can do. But the mind isn't built on simple binaries, and there is *another* opposite to anxiety: a deep sense of equanimity, an abiding sense of good and rightness in the world – the conviction that nothing can or will go wrong. It's a sense that has come to me unbidden from time to time, a gift from the universe – an unthinking, sweet feeling of ease that settled for a few weeks, then passed on. A state of grace, a glowing luminosity of the moment, as if music of transcendent harmony were playing just below the threshold of hearing, influencing body and mind.

But the converse has happened more often: periods of frenzy both socially and intellectually, when thoughts, ruminations and fears about the future succeeded one another with such rapidity that they wouldn't let me rest. Good sleep requires an ability to abandon yourself to the moment, and anxiety is its enemy. As I'd tumble exhausted into my bed my thoughts would whirl as quickly as ever; quicker, perhaps because of the lack of distractions. Every nudge towards the dreamy, disconnected images that precede sleep would cause me to jerk awake – too *conscious* of a process that should be intuitive and full of ease.

Daytime anxiety is often the price of night-time agitation – I might find myself worrying over possible futures, over past actions, over what colleagues or patients were thinking of me, over whether I'd turned off the hob at home, switched off the lights, left my keys hanging in the door. On the worst days, with no sleep overnight, I felt as if madness was circling me on black, leathery wings. The stink of it clung around me, lurching in fear at my belly. With each episode I became more accustomed to the feeling of anxiety in the body, and more able to register it as a sign that something had gone wrong – too much work, or too many obligations; not enough sleep, or not enough down time with friends and with family. I learned to see it as a warning to rethink my priorities, and settle any unresolved questions; I'd strayed into a perilous territory, and the most pressing concern was to get back on safe ground.

Mapmaking is a kind of magic: cartography takes the inconceivable complexity, plurality and diversity of the world and makes of it something comprehensible. A map is a model of reality, not reality itself – it is not the territory, and it is nothing like a photograph. Through my later teens I thought there was no greater ambition than to become a cartographer, and make sense of the world by mapping it. But then I fell in love with an atlas of anatomy, and decided to become a student not of geography, but of the body.

The body too is a kind of landscape, though the maps and models we make of it tend to take different names: 'anatomy', 'physiology' or 'biochemistry'. For the first couple of years of medical school I was obliged to learn the body's ways in health. In biochemistry I learned about the astonishing intricacy of the molecules and the chemical reactions that sustain life, and was daily stunned by the intimate machinery of even the simplest cells. In physiology I learned about the mechanics of the body – of blood pressures and pulses, of vital capacity and tissue elasticity, and learned to view health as a balance between competing forces – a creative tension of energies. In anatomy, with five others I cracked chests, exenterated pelvises, teased out the nerves and ganglia of the face. Over the course of the first year I had become enamoured of the anatomy's precision, order and elegance. I wanted to learn the names and forms of every muscle, bone, nerve and artery because that knowledge opened a new physical geography that was special because it *was* me: I carried it everywhere, and so did everyone else. It was like being inducted into a secret society dedicated to exploration of the geography of being. And in exploring that geography, my path kept returning me to the brain.

The French philosopher René Descartes became famous for his assertion 'I think therefore I am,' equating thought with existence, and at the same stroke insisting on a strict division between body and mind. *René* means 'born again' (a name which smacks of zealotry), while *Descartes* means 'of the maps'. Descartes' zealous and oversimplified map of the distinction between mind and body still influences much of medical science. He dissected dogs alive by nailing them to a board, convinced that their howls were mere reflex, and when he peered into a human brain decided that the soul was housed in the little gland between the cerebral hemispheres – the pineal gland (he was wrong: it makes melatonin, a hormone that shapes the rhythms of sleep and wakefulness).

Medicine in the twenty-first century believes it has moved on from Descartes, and in many ways it has. Yet in medicine we still use a very different map, when approaching problems of the mind, from the one used when attempting to understand the brain. The word *psychiatry*, concerned with problems of the mind, means 'doctoring of the soul', while *neurology*, concerned with problems of the brain, means 'knowledge of the nerves'. Yet for the last forty years much western psychiatry has behaved as if disorders of the mind are simply disorders of nerve function that we don't yet fully understand, as if our thinking is a simple matter of chemical levels in the brain. The truth is far more complicated.

★

To support myself through medical school I had two jobs: in term time I worked as a barman two nights a week: pulling pints, mopping spills and listening to the kinds of stories people tell when they're drunk. The bar was just around the corner from the city's High Court, and I'd often hear victorious tales of quashed convictions, as well as rueful accounts of guilty verdicts and unsuccessful appeals. It was good training for the practice of medicine, both for the instructive parables it offered as to the messy realities of addiction, and for the importance of cultivating neutral, compassionate listening skills.

For the other job I initially signed up with one of my professors to conduct an experiment on mouse brains, in the hope that mapping how they form in the embryo would help explain more about the development of human ones. In mice as in humans, after conception, one fertilised cell becomes two, then four, then eight, and so on, until a mass of cells implants into the lining of the womb and divides into three layers. The topmost embryonic layer of cells folds in on itself and sinks beneath the surface to form a tube that will eventually become the brain and spinal cord (it's the failure of this tube to close that causes the condition *spina bifida*, when the spinal cord doesn't submerge fully beneath the surface and remains tethered to the skin). So far so well-known, but what *wasn't* then understood was the order in which brain cells migrate to become different parts of the newborn brain. My job would be to help create a timed map of those brain cell migrations.

On the morning of my first day it was explained to me that my work would be to inject a chemical into the bellies of pregnant mice whose exact gestation was known. The chemical would embed itself into all the embryonic brain cells being created at that moment. Then, as soon as the baby mice were born, I was to kill them, slice up their brains and look under the microscope to see where those developing brain cells had finished up. It seemed the perfect job for an enthusiast of both maps and of neuroscience – a rare opportunity to contribute a pebble to the palace of scientific knowledge, and learn more about the brain, about laboratory work and about mapping the unknowns of the body. The only problem was, I couldn't bring myself to kill the mice.

The professor was short, neat, taciturn; he had a reputation for civility, and was rumoured to make all of his own clothes by hand. I was as surprised by my reluctance as he was: until arriving in that laboratory I had no idea that my reverence for life extended even to unborn lab mice. If life has in it something of the nature of a gift, then to slaughter those mice felt like an ungrateful exploitation of that gift.

The boss nodded in understanding as I apologised for having misled him: I shouldn't have accepted a job that involved injecting and slaughtering mice without considering more deeply whether I'd feel able, when the time came, to do just that. I supported, recognised and celebrated the value of the *knowledge* created by such work, but I just couldn't bring myself to do it. Disgraced and embarrassed I stumbled out of the lab. Not only had I disappointed the professor, and surely demolished any hope of a career in neuroscience, but I would also now be unemployed for the summer – and my rent was due. The neuroscience department looked out over a leafy Georgian square; I wondered whether I might be better suited to a career in tree surgery. Trees at least didn't wriggle when you tried to cut them open.

The rear of the department backed onto a warren of old Victorian buildings that housed the Anatomy department. I made my way through them, towards home, and in the corridor passed a friend who listened sympathetically, then pointed out a notice on a corkboard nearby. The Anatomy department was advertising a summer job, she said, and wanted six students to work in the dissection room, preparing specimens for the following academic year. I rerouted to the Anatomy office and signed up right away. I wouldn't spend my summer working on mouse brains, but on human ones.

The dissection room technician had been an undertaker before bringing his embalming skills to the university morgue. He was a kind, avuncular man of contradictions; he had been a soldier in the Territorial Army, and had recently returned from contributing to the first Gulf War. There was a bottle of whisky on his desk and he frequently offered drinks while we worked. I declined, but the bottle still needed replenishing every day; maybe he drank to get through the day long before his time in the Gulf, or maybe the war had driven him to it.

He spent much of his time in the Victorian brickwork basement preparing cadavers for dissection, and was always glad of company down there. I became adept at helping him hook up barrels of embalming fluid to the newly arrived bodies. Such a generous gift of people and their families – each body represented someone from the local community who had made a final offering of their own body to help students like me (and as a consequence, all the patients I'd ever see once qualified). The technician always said that he'd happily offer his own mortal remains to the department to become one of these 'silent teachers'. Too few years later, I heard that he did.

In most of the practice of medicine there's little in the way of hands-on craft. Unless you're a surgeon, or a pathologist, much work consists in listening to patient stories, sifting through the words they choose to convey the turmoil of their experience, and attending for clues and patterns. Most of diagnosis is in the patient's verbal account of their experience, not in examination findings. The great Edwardian physician William Osler supposedly summed this up as, 'Listen to the patient, they are trying to tell you the diagnosis.' A physical examination may refine your ideas: attending to sounds in the lungs, examining the belly or testing the nerves allows the doctor to compare their findings with a vast memory store of previous experiences examining others. Only then should you begin to draw your conclusions and formulate a plan for further tests and treatment, ideally together with the patient, ideally with wisdom and kindness.

But those summers spent as an anatomist gave me an insight into a different kind of life, one led by skill with the hands. Some would think of it as gruesome work, but it didn't feel like that – it felt like a privilege to be offered the time and space to deepen my knowledge of how the human body is put together. Every day was an education in glory: on arrival I'd switch on the radio, don an apron and gloves, unwrap the shrouds over the cadaver I was working on and begin the revelation.

Most of the nerves that give us bodily sensation, and that move our muscles, arise from the spinal cord; others that are involved in unconscious control of the body arise from the 'sympathetic trunks', running down the inside of the ribs at the back of the torso. But for much of the first summer I worked on dissections of what are known as the 'cranial nerves' – nerves that arise from, and feed directly into, the brain. There are twelve pairs of these: the first, the olfactory nerves, plug our sense of smell directly into one of the most primitive parts of our cerebrum. The cortex there is simpler than elsewhere (it has three layers instead of six), more ancient in terms of its evolution, and meshed into circuits that are active in memory and emotion (which is one reason why smells can be so evocative). The second, optic nerves, gives us sight – their fibres are thick and tough and, after fusing together an inch or two behind the bridge of the nose, they separate again and spray out in a broad radiation towards the visual cortex at the back of the brain. The third, fourth and sixth nerves move the eyeballs (three nerves might seem excessive, but then fine control of gaze is vital not only for tracking prey, avoiding predators, but also for signalling to others of our social group what is worth looking at). The fifth nerve gives us sensation to the face, as well as moving the muscles that chew. The seventh moves our muscles of facial expression (unique and particularly elegant, in that they're not attached to bone, but float freely within the soft tissues of the face*).

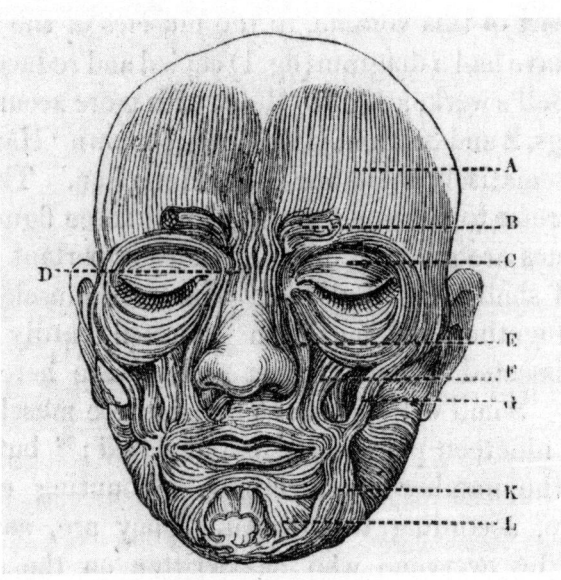

---

* The only other muscle in the human body like the muscles of facial expression is the one that moves the scrotum in men and, in women, the labia majora. Horses have a sheath of this kind of muscle over their whole body, which is why they can twitch the skin of their flanks and haunches.

The eighth gives us hearing and balance; the ninth and twelfth innervate the tongue and throat, while the eleventh stabilises the head on the neck. The tenth always seemed to me the most mysterious: termed 'the vagus', or 'wanderer', it exits near the base of the skull then meanders throughout the chest and abdomen, regulating, assessing, interpreting and controlling fundamental aspects of our being, from digestion to heart rate, the diameter of the airways of our lungs and the tightness of the muscles of our throat. The vagus nerve is proof of the link between states of mind and feelings of the body: there is as much information passed through it from body to brain as passes from brain to body. Each of these nerves had its own portal through the skull, and I pursued them to their origins as they emerged from the brain. It was through these channels that our perceptual world is created – not just the sensory one, but the emotional one too. The traffic through these nerves gives rise to feelings of anxiety and exhilaration, fear and torpor: they are the reason why anxiety makes our throat, jaw and chest tight, but our bowels loose; why terror makes our hearts hammer and our limbs tremble.

It wasn't until the end of my second summer as an anatomist that I created my finest dissection: the knot of unconscious nerve fibres, millimetres behind the eye, that governs weeping.* What better proof of there being no true distinction between mind and body, or that the mind is itself embodied, than this tangle of nerves where thought or feeling becomes water – a transformation as astonishing as water into wine?

Anatomy had dazzled me with its elegance and intricacy, but as I went on in the work the emergence of consciousness,

---

* The pterygopalatine ganglion.

manifest as a self, began to feel the greater miracle. There was a cell, and then there were lots of cells, some sensory nerves, some motor nerves with muscles, and some connections in between, and – hey presto! – a fully functional mind *and* self, in dynamic interaction. *Being* emerged from the interaction between a bunch of cells (but what a bunch!) and its environment, in a dynamic whirlpool of energy and possibility. For a mind to emerge from matter, as my own seemed to have done, seemed like an astonishingly unlikely event – it felt equally absurd both that the mind emerges from the firing of neurons, and that it does not. The miracle made both unthinkable.

I began to see how habitual states of mind become written on the body. I remember a muscled male cadaver with shaved head, his arms sleeved with prison tattoos. The left ventricle of his heart was thickened from untreated high blood pressure, and I wondered how many years of stress he'd endured. His aorta was tortured and brittle – a smoker, for sure, with a poor diet, sucking on tobacco and greasy food as a lifelong substitute for something else he lacked. His lungs were grey, reticulated with black soot and tobacco tar, outlining in the channels of his lymph all the residues that he had inhaled – I wondered too if he had ever worked as a miner. Beneath the layers of his face I discovered the muscles which lift the angles of our mouths into a smile were for him withered and frail, while those that pull those corners down into a frown were strong and thick – evidence that this had been a man who smiled rarely, but often had cause to frown.

It was barely fathomable that the brain and all the nerves I dissected had begun sixty or so years earlier as a clot of stem cells when this man had been an embryo. I opened the top of his skull to look down on his brain floating in a nutritive bath of shock-absorbing fluid – the box of delights that had been home to every experience of his late existence. After the brain's removal, with care I laid open the fluid-filled chambers that bathed its core. The paired lateral ventricles, one at the centre of each cerebral hemisphere, were united at the third ventricle along the brain's midline. The third ventricle rinses the lower reaches of brain all the way down to its most primitive elements – those responsible for growth, fertility, blood pressure, sleeping and waking.

QVINTA SEPTIMI LIBRI FIGVRA·

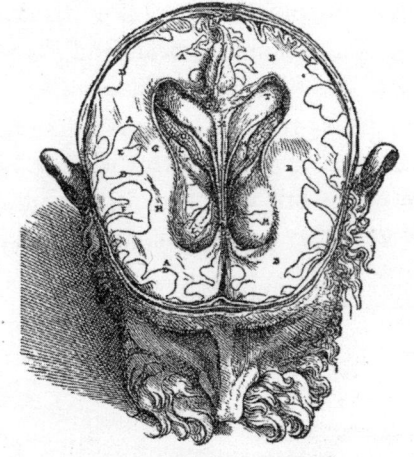

PRAESENS figura quòd ad relictam in caluaria cerebri portionē attinet, nulla ex parte uariat: atꝗ id foli habet proprium, quod callosum corpus hic anteriori sua se de à cerebro primùm liberauimus, ac dein eleuatum in posteriora refleximus, septum dextri ac sinistri uentriculorum di uellentes, & corporis instar testudinis extruct superiorem superficiem ob oculos ponētes. Ab A A, A, A itaꝗ & B, B, ad Q B, ac dein D, D, D, & E & F, & G & H eadem hic indicant, quæ in quarta figura. Sic quoque & L, L, & M, M, & O & P & Q eadem insinuant. R, R, R *Notatur inferior callosi corporis superficies. est enim id à sua sede motum, atque in posteriora reflexum.*

S,T,V Supe·

The lateral ventricles were first described by a Greek-Egyptian anatomist, Herophilus, who noticed that a ribbon of scarlet tissue along each one which generates cerebrospinal fluid resembled parts of the placenta (Greek: *chorion*), and named it accordingly – he called it the 'choroid plexus'. In each wing of the third ventricle there was a circular opening named for a genius anatomist of the Edinburgh Enlightenment, Alexander Monro, who had worked in the same department that now employed me. With a halved brain in my hands I could peer through those openings as if through a keyhole, and wonder at how this kilo or two of tissue could effect such a magical transformation, of matter into consciousness, or consciousness refracting through matter, a transformation that even today resists explanation.

One day I would have to make decisions about others' lives based on how well I could visualise this galaxy of complexity under the skin – the routes traced by arteries and nerves as they wind miraculously through the cosmos of the body, the precise location of organs, muscles and bones, the important constellations and shapes of it, and the smaller, more beautiful and intricate ones. The mystery of the brain. It was a privilege to work each day with my hands, asked to be creative not with the stuff of the earth – with metal, or clay – but with this other stuff, the substance of people who've grown and lived and loved and died.

2

CONSTELLATIONS OF THE MIND

Those who first invented and then named the
constellations were storytellers. Tracing an
imaginary line between a cluster of stars gave them
an image and an identity.

John Berger

Someone is shot, and almost dies; the fragility of life is pain-
fully and intimately revealed to him. He goes on to have
flashbacks of the event, finds that he can no longer relax or
enjoy himself; his sleep is restless, agitated and unrefreshing.
His relationships suffer, and wither, as he is progressively disturbed and distressed by intrusive memories of the event.

This could read as a description of many patients I've seen
in clinic and in the emergency room over the years, suffering
what has in recent decades been called PTSD, or post-traumatic stress disorder. But it isn't one of my patients; it's a
description of Maricha, uncle of Ravana, recounted in the
7,000-year-old Indian epic *The Ramayana*.

Other ancient epics describe textbook cases of what we
now call 'generalised anxiety disorder', with excessive fear
and rumination, loss of focus and inability to sleep. Others
again describe what sounds like suicidal depression. Mental
suffering has been with human beings for as long as human
beings have experienced mental life, but the names and

labels we give its manifestations are always evolving.

For over twenty years now my work has been as a general practitioner ('GP'). Professional psychiatrists are today so taken up with managing extreme mental illness that much of a GP's work concerns the everyday unhappiness, anxiety and sorrows that blunt and blight a life without threatening it – the many miseries of living that never make it to the door of a psychiatrist. In the UK specialist psychiatrists are known as 'consultants' because GPs like me can 'consult' them for advice, but the ultimate responsibility for care usually remains with the GP. We are more than our fleeting feelings, but our mental states are where we live, they filter every experience and sensation. The mind creates the world we inhabit, and profoundly influences bodily health: psychiatry, then, is a fundamental part of every consultation I have. Thirty years in medicine has shown me just how hard life can be for many people. It has also taught me not to make too fine a distinction between suffering of the body and mind.

When I worked in emergency medicine I frequently had the sense of being witness to a defining moment of someone's life: a car crash, a heart attack, a brain haemorrhage. There is never much latitude in how to approach such crises – there are few options, because life-saving protocols must be adhered to. But in general practice I learned that there was great freedom in how to approach each consultation; the manner of being and engaging with the patient was intricately interconnected with outcome, and was part of the therapy. There was more scope to personalise the treatment of each patient. The Hungarian psychoanalyst Michael Balint called it 'the doctor as the drug'.

Doctors continually practise psychological therapy in the way they approach their patients, break bad news, instil optimism or pessimism, foster autonomy or a feeling of helplessness. Between a third and a half of the patients who book an appointment with me do so in the hope of relieving some problem that touches on their mental health. Every day I'm given new examples of the many paths people take through life, seeking happiness or success. No two days are the same, and every encounter brings reflections on the challenges and rewards of being human.

I've met people in their eighties who, through our conversations in the consulting room, have realised that the root of their unhappiness is a sense of having been unmothered as an infant, almost a century before. I've met others who have come to realise their overeating, or obsessive cleaning, or alcoholism, are attempts to fill an emptiness which could be more reliably filled in other, healthier ways, and also has its origins in childhood experiences. At birth each of us embarked on an adventure into an ocean of possibilities. Some find themselves in tranquil, benign and relatively sheltered waters, while others meet storms, reefs and dangerous undercurrents as soon as they're born. Sometimes I realise the patient isn't necessarily looking for a cure, but for validation of their suffering, a listening ear, or a sense of fellowship. Sometimes it's not possible to identify why someone's mind has tipped into anxiety, depression or psychosis, but there are usually some clues to at least part of what has brought them to such a frightening place, and it's usually possible to offer some guidance as to how to begin finding a way out. One of the many rewards of practising medicine is the way it enables you to walk through social divides, welcomed equally at bedsides in slums and in mansions, as at home in an elite research university as in a humble community clinic. Another is how it requires creativity of approaches: from objective to subjective, from paternalistic to maternalistic, from didactic to collaborative.

Conscious experience is a flowing, dynamic river of influences; the mind's topography of possibility is always changing. It can't but help be in a state of flux – sometimes dominated by memory, sometimes by anticipation, sometimes by immediate perceptions – which means that it can be nudged, in its changes, towards health – which means 'wholeness'. The mental fields of experience shimmer with dynamism, becoming narrow or expansive, colourful or monotone. Some people stay in roughly level mental fields their whole lives, while others move between radically exotic states of mind. It can feel as if, though I sit in the consulting room, I'm a voyager of the minds and stories of my patients.

'Life is inherently difficult,' wrote the English psychiatrist and paediatrician Donald Winnicott, and 'it follows that in everyone there will be symptoms, any one of which, under certain conditions, could be a symptom of illness. Even the most kindly, understanding background of home-life cannot alter the fact that ordinary human development is hard'. When the feelings that filter through into our awareness are negative, then clinicians call them 'symptoms'. When those feelings are positive, we tend to regard them simply as elements of well-being.

Our states of mind can make prisoners of us, make us want to die, make us slash at our own bodies or make us believe we're immortal or invulnerable. They can torment us with visions and persecutory voices, and distort the way we see our own bodies and those of others. They can make it impossible for us to sleep, sink us in addictions, make us incapable of focus, self-control or contentment. They can destroy our families, make it impossible for us to communicate, to love, to be part of the very communities that would help sustain us. Just about any aspect of mental life can go wrong, and how we characterise and make sense of those disturbances has huge implications for how we find our way back to a sense of ease.

It has become routine to talk about mental suffering as

caused by discrete mental disorders, as if the labels we give those kinds of suffering had the same empirical and verifiable reality as any disease. Many people now use the words 'mental health' as interchangeable with 'mental illness' – as in, 'I'm here for my mental health, doctor.' The ubiquity of this kind of language has destigmatised emotional and mental distress, encouraged sufferers to seek help, fostered communities of others with similar problems and neutralised much of the guilt formerly associated with such difficulties. But medical words are powerful, and medical labels can become self-fulfilling spells that curse as often as they cure. As Esmé Weijun Wang writes in her memoir of schizoaffective disorder (a type of psychosis in which mood swings are prominent): 'My new diagnosis bore no curative function, but it did imply that to be high-functioning would be difficult, if not impossible, for me.' And as Dr Benji Waterhouse, a British NHS psychiatrist (and stand-up comedian), puts it, 'Sometimes I wonder if the medical-sounding diagnoses, clusters and codes that I'm forced to enter on endless forms couldn't more honestly be replaced by "NFI" (no fucking idea), "SLS" (shit-life syndrome) or "PNA" (pretty normal actually).'

Though many terms we use to describe mental illness have no reliable basis other than consensus among a committee of doctors, I've known people whose lives have taken on utterly different destinies, good and bad, solely from being given the label of a new diagnosis. But in recent years I've encountered more people with the unfounded conviction that these labels have a fixed reality, that they are based on hard evidence, and that they therefore confer some kind of fate. Sometimes among those same patients I encounter increasing disquiet with mental health labelling, and a rising awareness that such labels can become self-reinforcing. Many recipients of those labels are beginning to question the authority on which they're based. Trends in psychiatry reflect trends in society more broadly, but the authority for determining what constitutes mental illness remains with committees of specialists. In this book I hope to make a plea for greater flexibility and humility in how we think about the mind, and challenge aspects of that authority. I'd like us to hold those labels more lightly, and with more hope.

The subject is important, because the twenty-first century is seeing an epidemic of mental ill health, at least according to the terms of how modern psychiatry defines it. A recent survey of a thousand young people in the UK found over two-thirds believed they have, or have had, a mental disorder. We are broadening the criteria for what counts as illness at the same time as lowering the thresholds for diagnosis. As long ago as 2008 a study found that in the United States half of the population would, across their lifetimes, meet criteria for a mental illness. A quarter of the population was found to be suffering one at any one time, according to the then-current edition of the *Diagnostic and Statistical Manual of the American Psychiatric Association* (DSM-IV), often thought of as the bible of western psychiatry (though in truth it has evolved into a billing manual for US healthcare, and was never intended to set out ultimate truths about the mind).

It's been almost twenty years since then; reported problems are increasing. The *DSM-5* of 2013 broadened the net of what counts as a psychiatric disorder still further (the shift away from Roman numerals from 'IV' to '5' was deliberate). Other classification systems have been revised and enlarged: in Europe it's more common to use instead the *ICD* or *International Classification of Diseases* and in east Asia the *Chinese Classification of Mental Disorders*. Also in use are a Japanese Clinical Modification of *ICD*, the *Cuban Glossary of Psychiatry* and the *Latin American Guide for Psychiatric Diagnosis* – all have been revised and enlarged in recent years.

Maps of the world are not the territory, and maps of the mind such as the *DSM* and *ICD* are only models of how to think about thinking. They are instruments, only useful to the extent that they help us ease suffering, and meet the many challenges of being and staying alive.

Jean-Paul Sartre called emotion 'a magical transformation of the world', and its magic can be a dark one. Imagine for a moment life falling into monochrome. Laughter and smiles become forced, mechanical and, eventually, impossible. There seems to be no beauty in art, in nature, and even music loses its power. Everything and everyone is dull, brutish and graceless, and there seems no elegance, opportunity or excitement in the world. It's the night-side of life: cumbersome, decrepit, sluggish and gloomy. I've known people for whom episodes of depression cast a dark cloak of paranoia around each of their relationships, draining the joy out of seeing family, of friends, and attacking motivation, ambition and everything in which they once took pleasure.

It's a surprising truth that science still doesn't understand how such shifts in mood are governed – neither the changeable spirits of mind that come and go from day to day, nor those background moods that move slowly, often imperceptibly, over months and even years. If feelings come and go like weather, then our background temperament can be imagined as something more stable, like climate. But climate, as we are all now perilously aware, is quite capable of changing too.

Although the suffering caused by mental problems is as grave as any kind of physical suffering, and can sometimes be life-threatening, a glance at history confirms that the frameworks we use to understand it change with the times. The word 'emotion' was only invented in the 1830s;* before

---

* By Thomas Brown, a professor of philosophy at Edinburgh.

that it was more common to speak of 'sentiments', 'spirits' or even 'humours'. And around the world different cultures view the derangements of the mind in utterly different ways, sometimes with better consequences: for example, if you had a choice where to be diagnosed with schizophrenia you wouldn't choose the West, where outcomes are statistically poorer than in other parts of the world. Shekhar Saxena, a former director of mental health for the World Health Organisation and now a professor of global mental health at Harvard, said he would rather get a diagnosis of schizophrenia in Ethiopia or Sri Lanka than in the West, because there's a greater chance in those countries of being able to carve out a niche in life that makes space for your symptoms, of your life continuing to have meaning, of being able to make sense of your experience, of remaining connected to community. In West Africa I once visited a tree near the heart of a village where people who became psychotic were chained up until they recovered. It sounds barbaric, until you reflect that for some people being chained to the right tree, in the heart of your community, with the right people checking in on you, might conceivably work out better than being locked up in a distant psychiatric clinic staffed by overworked strangers.

As human beings we are bathed in language; we rely on it to make sense of the world, and different languages and cultures take different approaches to thinking, feeling and being. Some kinds of distress I'll touch on in this book seem common to every era and culture, while others arise and fall away, shapeshifting under the influence of society and community. The American psychotherapist Clarissa Pinkola Estés summarised just a few alternative ways her clients had described their mental states to her over the years, as distinct from the lists of labels in the psychiatry textbooks:

dry, fatigued, frail, depressed, confused, gagged, muzzled, unaroused. Feeling frightened, halt or weak, without inspiration, without animation, without soulfulness, without meaning, shame-bearing, chronically fuming, volatile, stuck, uncreative, compressed, crazed. Feeling powerless, chronically doubtful, shaky, blocked, unable to follow through, giving one's creative life over to others, life-sapping choices in mates, work or friendships, suffering to live outside one's own cycles, overprotective of self, inert, uncertain, faltering, inability to pace oneself or set limits.

It's a rich inventory of possibility, immediately recognisable for those of us who live with the realities of getting along in life, and very different from the clinical lists found in any textbook. Pinkola Estés recognised that trying to force her clients' experiences into a rigid, monotone map of the *DSM* would dishonour the richness of their experiences – and wouldn't necessarily help them to get better.

I knew a sailor once whose knowledge of the stars meant that, wherever he was in the world, he could look up and feel at home. Doctors speak of 'constellations' of symptoms, as if the body were a galaxy, and the process of diagnosis simply the imposition of stories upon the patterns of nature, the way we may look at a pattern of stars and see Cassiopeia, or the Great Bear.*

When working as a doctor in India, or in Africa, I've often thought the same of physical medicine – that pneumonia, liver failure or meningitis follow very similar patterns and give similar signs wherever you are in the world. But the mind

---

* 'Constellation of symptoms' first appeared in the *Lancet* in 1887, to describe the diffuse presentation of kidney disease.

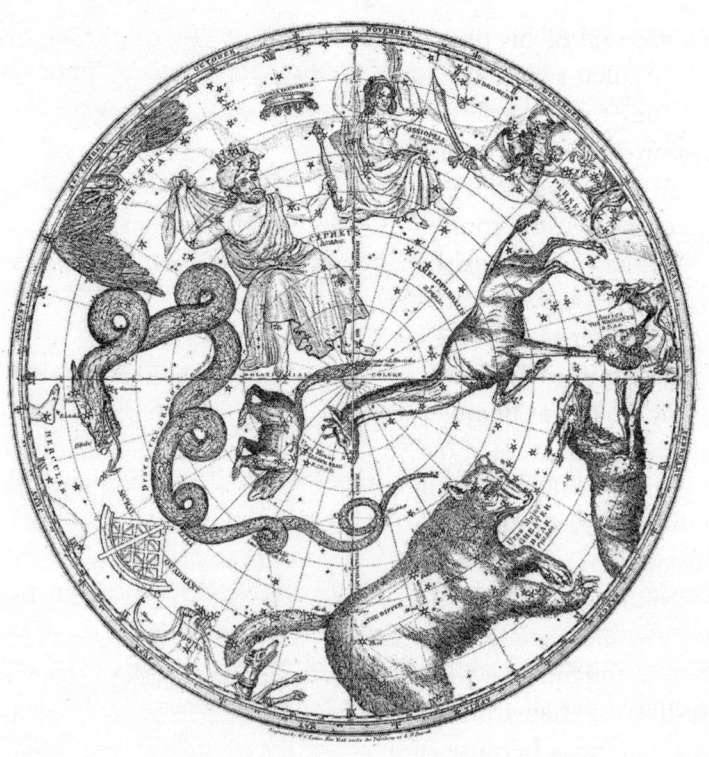

is different, inextricably cultural; each society elucidates singular arrangements from its disturbances. Those alternative patterns are just as valid, and remain useful to guide navigation across the mind's territory. For some people, lost in a joyless, frightening or anxious realm of the mind, it might be necessary to draw a new map to help them reorientate their surroundings and find their way to safety. The Italian psychiatrist Paolo Milone described this beautifully: 'Every psychiatrist, with every single one of his patients, forms a separate universe, a separate stellar system, in which the same laws of physics apply, but with different masses, velocities, orbits, gravitations, atmospheres.' The therapist Carl Rogers, famous for his stance of unconditional positive regard for his clients, said of his time in the consulting room that 'There is a peculiar satisfaction in really hearing someone: it is like listening to the music of the spheres' – as if psychotherapy is a comparable activity to stargazing.

At medical school I too was taught to understand mental experiences using constellations of symptoms that point to a particular mental health diagnosis – depression, generalised anxiety, obsessive-compulsiveness, attention-deficit, schizo-phrenia. But as a GP seeing patients at the milder end of the spectrum of mental suffering, what I saw in clinic was not a set of labels but unique blends of strengths and vulnerabili-ties, with vast areas of overlap between different conditions. I began to see how suffering of the mind exists in thousands of gradations, from minor unhappiness to suicidal depression, say, or from mildly suspicious to psychotically paranoid. One person might have withdrawn to their bed, unable to leave the house, because of a paralysing crash in their mood, while another might have withdrawn because of terror over what lay beyond their front door. One person might have devel-oped anorexia because of an obsessiveness over food itself, or thinness, while another developed it because a traumatic, abusive childhood left a legacy of need to control what goes in and out of the body.

I began to appreciate more fully how just a little of some traits such as obsessiveness or elation or rumination could be helpful, while an excess usually ended up being harmful – it's an ancient idea that virtue or excellence lies not in extremes, but in balance. A little anxiety is a good thing – it keeps us safe – but if it starts to take over we need to find ways to roll it back and keep it in check. Our minds' capacity for delu-sion and hallucination hints at something fundamental to our humanity – our openness to creative reinterpretations of reality. But when that capacity becomes unmoored, it can destroy a life – and often does (psychotic illness, when the fabric of reality itself becomes distorted and unreliable, has a higher suicide rate than depression).

Someone with a tendency to elation and disinhibition can be a boon for any community – we need some rule-breakers and utopian dreamers who believe themselves to be capable of anything. But when those feelings tip over into mania it often wrecks families, friendships and livelihoods. A pupil with ADHD might be challenging for a teacher trying to control a boisterous classroom, but the energy, enthusiasm and multitasking associated with such tendencies can also be a blessing. And what is low mood except the excruciating awareness that life could and indeed should feel better than it does? Every mental health problem I see in clinic has at its core a tendency that, in a more measured dose, or different context, could contribute to human well-being, rather than detract from it. If we were able to hold the labels more lightly, aware of the human tendencies they oversimplify, would we be able to create a society more accepting of difference? Might it be less stigmatising, but also more hopeful, and more open to recovery? Our current labels pretend to certainties that, when you scrape the surface of the science behind them, they have no claim to.

Maps of the mind and the labels we apply to them are subject to change as cultures evolve; we mustn't give those labels more weight than they are able to bear. If the stories those constellations tell are unhelpful, we can redraw them; if they show promise, we can elaborate them. Physicians with wisdom know that they don't have all the answers; they leave room for doubt, for new thinking, and for telling creative new stories about the life of the mind. And what other kind of life is there?

3

PHYSICIANS, PRIESTS AND PROPHECY

It is the history of our kindnesses that alone makes
this world tolerable.

Robert Louis Stevenson

The earliest healers we know of in history were in ancient
Mesopotamia. There were three kinds: the seer or prophet
(*bârû*) who would predict outcomes, the priest (*âshipu*) who
could perform incantations and exorcise demons, and the
physician (*âsû*), whose expertise was in potions and wound
care. By the time of the pharaohs of Egypt, ways of healing
had proliferated. Herodotus wrote of Egyptian physicians,
'some attend to the disorders of the eyes, others to those of
the head, some take care of the teeth, others are conversant
with all diseases of the bowels.' Mental distress was the prov-
ince of the priest, but other physicians had a hand in the
maintenance of aspects of well-being. Egyptians thought the
heart was the seat of consciousness, but at least one Egyptian military surgeon noticed that a blow to the head can
strike someone dumb, and that a broken neck can cause you
to lose control of your bladder.

Ancient Egypt was a proctologist's dream: the body
was seen as a river system that, like the Nile, had to be kept
flowing. If it blocked, mental and physical suffering would
result. Ancient Egyptians devoted three days every month

to the clearing of their intestines by enemas, purgatives and emetics, to flush out 'rotten' contents that were believed to cause illness. Peace of mind required a peaceful bowel. One of the most privileged positions at court was Keeper of the Royal Rectum.

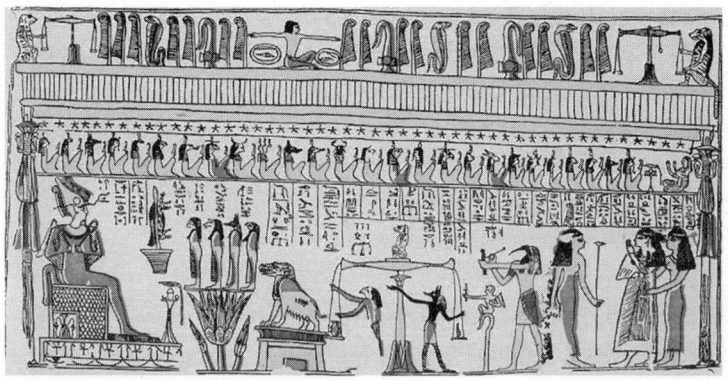

Some ideas keep coming back around. In the early twentieth century ancient ideas about the bowel's relation to health resurfaced in Chicago, with an American homeopath-turned-surgeon by the name of Bayard Holmes, who became convinced that madness was caused by toxins in the gut. Holmes developed a procedure whereby the appendix was brought up to the surface of the skin then used as a conduit to flush a daily cleansing irrigation through the colon. When Holmes's own son Ralph developed psychosis in 1916, he operated. Ralph died four days later from complications of surgery.

My own medical training in the late twentieth century was dismissive of the bowel's influence on the mind, and yet now, thirty years on, it's evident that there are as many neurons in the human gut as there are in the brain of a dog, there are more bacteria inside our intestines than we have cells in our bodies, and that the messages sent *to* our brains from the gut are as important as the messages received *from* the brain. Gut health affects mental health; 'gut feelings' are real, and can sometimes be a better guide to decision-making than what is consciously or rationally perceived, because they're informed by subconscious intuition. After decades of practice I'm starting to think the Egyptians might have been onto something; I pay as much attention to the prescription of laxatives as I do antidepressants.

The *Iliad* and the *Odyssey* are thought to have been written down around 800 BCE, and conjure a world of divine inspiration and retribution, of furies and fates, noticeable for the humanity of their character portraits and sensitivity to disturbances of the mind. Ajax, caught up in a frenzy of rageful grief, attacks a flock of sheep after becoming deluded into believing them enemies. Achilles is manifestly a traumatised soldier, enslaved by overwhelming fantasies of pride, lust and revenge. On the island of the Lotus Eaters Odysseus encounters a drugged, drop-out community of substance-misusing addicts. The psychosis, trauma, addiction, depression recognised by Homer could read as a case list from one of my own clinics. The characters in the *Iliad* see gods and hear voices: there's a view that the capacity to hear voices is a primitive and important part of our humanity, and that auditory hallucinations reveal an earlier, less rational version of ourselves.

The doctor described in Homer's the *Iliad* is Aesculapius, a kind of tribal chieftain-medic. Later sources transform him into a god. His temples were early hospitals where sufferers in body or mind sought cures in rituals heavy with symbolism. They took draughts of sedative drugs and slept in chambers alongside holy snakes that, with their venom and their shedding skin, were considered emblematic of renewal. The visions and dreams that resulted, the drama of the setting, the faith and mystery of the event, and no doubt some helpful listening and advice from the physician-priests who staffed the temples, would point the way towards a cure.

Aristotle, the great systematiser and observer of the world, was the son of a doctor. He touched on issues of mental health when he emphasised his doctrine of virtue being the avoidance of excess: health resided in moderation in all things. In his book *De Anima* ('Of the Soul') he grasped the central difficulty of understanding states of mind when we are largely ignorant as to how they relate to states of the body. Psyche means 'soul': Aristotle asked whether psychological distress is a product of some material change in the body, or of the ethereal flux of the soul. 'This', he wrote in response, 'it is necessary to grasp, but not easy ... Grasping anything trustworthy concerning the soul is completely and in every way among the most difficult of affairs.' Neurophilosophy and neuropsychology remain 'the most difficult of affairs' today. We still don't have the slightest idea how consciousness really works. The *International Dictionary of Psychology* (written by Stuart Sutherland) notoriously has the following wry but candid entry on the subject: 'Consciousness is a fascinating but elusive phenomenon; it is impossible to specify what it is, what it does, or why it evolved. Nothing worth reading has been written on it.'

Mental health for the Greeks and Romans was dependent on the balance of four humours: blood, phlegm, black bile and yellow bile, as well as a life-giving force of *pneuma*, or breath. As a system it has parallels in traditional Indian and Chinese medicine, preoccupied as they are with flows of energies, with the life-giving forces of *prana* and *chi* respectively. An excess of the four humours was later proposed as an explanation of four personality types – a classification so useful as a framework for understanding human behaviour that it has survived into the twenty-first century: melancholic (depressed), phlegmatic (resilient), sanguine (cheerful) and choleric (angry). Like all good maps or models its usefulness does not mean that it is *true*.

Treatment of mental illness was about recognising which humour was overabundant, and correcting the imbalance with diet, exercise, purgatives and bleeding. The story of humours persisted for almost 2,000 years because of its great explanatory power, and its potential to be modified for almost any situation – allowing physicians to backtrack when their predictions went wrong.

Before we dismiss the idea of humours determining our mood or character, it's noticeable that the 'neurotransmitter hypothesis' of mental illness, whereby depression was for many decades deemed to arise from a lack of serotonin, is a modern manifestation of the same idea. When I was a medical student much study was focused on drugs that effected their actions at the level of the synapses between brain cells, thought to take effect by either stimulating or blocking the excitation or inhibition of brain cell firing. Now it's known that the function of synapses is far more complex than presumed, and that they may switch sides, so to speak: an excitatory synapse can pivot to become inhibitory, and vice versa. We don't understand how they do this, or how the medications we use to manage mental distress influence this process. We struggle still to define brain function at the level of a single cell, never mind a teeming network of billions of them.

For a few decades some sufferers and clinicians found the idea that mood was determined by levels of chemicals in the brain a useful shorthand explanation, and there's evidence that some drugs can, over years of use, influence the depletion of some neurotransmitters (e.g. long-term amphetamine use for ADHD may diminish the dopamine content of the brain). But the idea of neurotransmitter excess or deprivation as a cause of mental illness is wrong-headed – like thinking you could fix a car engine solely by manipulating the supply of petrol. It is now, thankfully, being discarded into the dustbin of human ideas.

The *DSM-5* has the following entry for mania:

> Decreased need for sleep, more talkative than usual or pressure to keep talking, flight of ideas or subjective experience that thoughts are racing, attention too easily drawn to unimportant or irrelevant external stimuli, increase in goal-directed activity (either socially, at work or school, or sexually).

Compare this with a list compiled by the Roman physician Soranus (*c.* 100 CE) of the causes and consequences of mania:

> Continual sleeplessness, excesses of venery, anger, grief, anxiety or superstitious fear, a shock or blow, intense straining of the senses and the mind in study, business, or other ambitious pursuits.

Passages like these give me a kind of historical vertigo; they demonstrate that although science and society are always in evolution, certain aspects of our humanity appear to be changeless, and the symptoms of mania are constant across the centuries. Between the physicians of the early Roman Empire and those of the European Middle Ages there was little progress on ideas of mental health, until a Swiss physician called Paracelsus began to throw out all the old learning, declaring it almost useless. In contrast to the prevailing orthodoxy that medicine was to be learned from books, he wrote, 'I have not been ashamed to learn from tramps, butchers and barbers.' His riddling, paradox-strewn writings teeter on a three-way fulcrum between the medieval, mystical and modern. He was an alchemist but also a doctor, an army medic who went on campaigns with Venetian soldiers to Russia and Egypt, who not only rejected the idea of the four humours but also declared the learned professors of the great European medical schools to be ignorant. As a piece of paradigm-shifting theatre he once set fire to the canonical works of Galen, the Roman founder of the western medical tradition.

Like a priest, he also insisted that the most important principle at work in his profession was love,* maintaining that the best physicians nourish a love for both the profession and their patients. He was alive to the transformative effect of optimism and belief: 'Physicians should not hold the effect of curses as nonsense, you have no inkling of the power and might of the will,' he wrote – a position now being proven again, in the twenty-first century, by studies into the formidable power of placebos. The science writer Shankar Vedantam reported in the *Washington Post* more than twenty years ago that 'After thousands of studies, hundreds of millions of prescriptions and tens of billions of dollars in sales, two things are certain about pills that treat depression: antidepressants like Prozac, Paxil and Zoloft work. And so do sugar pills.' Placebos that you have to pay handsomely for work better than cheap ones, capsules seem to work better than tablets, and coloured capsules work better than white or clear ones. Blue and greens capsules work better as sedatives, while pinks and reds work better as stimulants and painkillers. Size matters too: it seems that we trust either tiny pills or big ones

---

* Oliver Sacks, in *Awakenings*, wrote on this theme: 'Eros is the oldest and strongest of the gods; that love is the *alpha* and *omega* of being; and that the work of healing, of rendering whole, is first and last, the business of love.'

(the latter because they're more impressive, and the former presumably because tiny capsules must contain powerful drugs).

The first systematic attempt at a cartography of the mind was undertaken a couple of centuries after Paracelsus, in France. François Boissier de Sauvages de Lacroix was a contemporary of Linnaeus, the Swedish botanist who created the taxonomy of life that is still used today. (It is thanks to Linnaeus that we are *Homo sapiens*, 'thinking' or 'wise' man; though Linnaeus recognised that biologically speaking there was little to separate humanity from the apes, he felt he had to give us a separate genus: 'if I had called man an ape, or vice versa,' he wrote, 'I would have fallen under the ban of all the ecclesiastics. It may be that as a naturalist I ought to have done so.')

Sauvages was a physician in Montpellier, a medical centre renowned throughout Europe for the depth and subtlety of its botany – an emphasis inherited from the medieval Arab world, which had preserved and elaborated much Greek learning while Europe was stuck in the Dark Ages. In 1763 he published *Nosologia Methodica*, a classification of illness that was explicitly inspired by Linnaeus's system for the classification of plants. There were to be ten major classes of illness, and the eighth of these was 'madness', which was divided into genera and also into species. A year later in 1764 Voltaire was able to write, in his *Dictionnaire philosophique*: 'Insanity: A brain disease that keeps a man from thinking and acting as other men do. If he cannot take care of his property he is put under tutelage; if his behaviour is unacceptable, he is isolated; if he is dangerous, he is confined; if he is furious, he is tied.' From the late seventeenth century up until the Battle of Waterloo, the entrance to London's Bedlam Hospital was topped by two statues: one representing Melancholy, and one Mania ('Raving Madness'). These

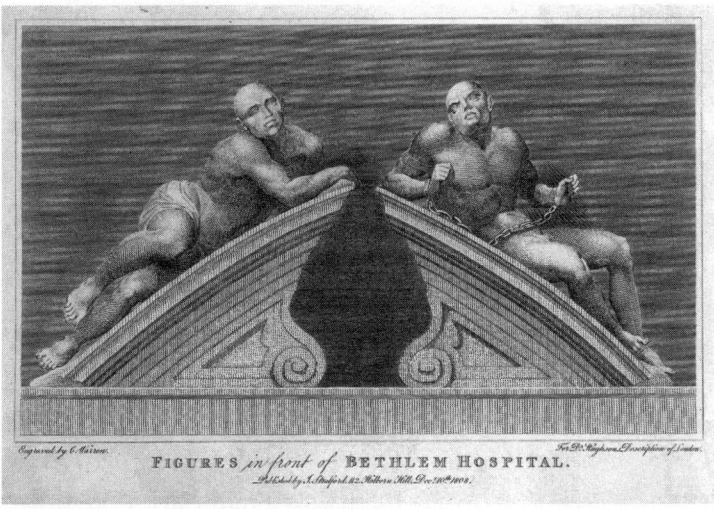

FIGURES *in front of* BETHLEM HOSPITAL.

were the two simple stars in the firmament of feeling to which all human distress was related.

Like those anonymous storytellers who first named the constellations, putting stars into patterns and shapes that made sense for them, physicians with a special interest in derangements of the mind attempted to discern patterns in the anguish of their patients, to help orientate and steer them through the storms of life. Those blunt distinctions evolved over the following two centuries into the lists found in the *DSM* and *ICD*. The first American asylum manual, the forerunner to the *DSM*, was published in 1918; it had evolved from Bedlam's two presiding maladies to a grand total of twenty-two potential diagnoses. The latest manifestation has over 400 separate categories of mental disorder. A worrying development is the expansion of the manual to include categories of *risk* of developing a particular state of mind, each as a separate condition. We're all at risk of all sorts of things – it's a shift that, if extended further, could find pathology in all of us.

A materialist belief that mental distress *is* brain disease didn't preclude some early psychiatrists from bringing a compassionate and humane perspective to bear. In the 1840s John Connolly of the Hanwell Asylum outside London resolved *not* to restrain his patients; he showed in his case summaries a remarkable sensitivity to the mental and social life of each individual. He was also a phrenologist: someone who believed that the brain held within it discrete lumps of matter responsible for different mental attributes, and that the swelling or diminution of those attributes would be reflected in the shape of the overlying skull, a theory later enthusiastically embraced by racists. As an approach to understanding the mind and body it seems ridiculous now, a reminder that medical science often gets things wrong. But just as the neurotransmitter hypothesis was a recasting of the old idea of the four humours, so phrenology is not too distant from our current obsession with brain scans and the way they 'light up', depending on mental states, activities and tendencies. That view is already being mocked as an unsophisticated oversimplification – a busy bit of brain is as likely to be inhibiting something as it is to be doing something, and the more expert or accomplished someone is at a task, the less brain activity is seen when they engage in it.

In the later nineteenth century the cutting edge of new thinking of the mind was in German academic circles, and the most celebrated of its neuropsychiatrists was a Prussian, Carl Wernicke, who sought to understand the link between brain and mind by unpicking the relationship between sound and meaning, words and understanding. He'd noticed that when people sustained damage to a certain brain region, now known as 'Wernicke's area', they could speak but could not read, or understand speech. For Wernicke the brain was an organ for making associations between words and things in a dynamic, complicated and ever-evolving way. 'The soul', he said rather beautifully, 'is the sum of all possible associations.'

Around the same time psychiatrists began peering into the idiosyncrasies of human sexuality. A Viennese physician called Richard von Krafft-Ebing published his *Psychopathia Sexualis* in 1866, setting out his view, for example, that homosexuality was a constitutional degeneration. Other writers were more nuanced: his near contemporary Axel Munthe, a Swedish doctor who trained in Paris, was a mesmerising, charismatic fabulist in addition to his gifts as a thinker on the hinterlands of the mind. He had great success as a popular doctor to a wealthy clientele in Paris and in Rome. He defended homosexuality in a way that seems lukewarm by today's standards, but by the standards of his own time it was revolutionary. He counselled strongly against the idea that sexuality could be 'treated': 'energetic interference often does more harm than good,' he wrote of the men who had come to him *asking* for conversion therapy; 'they are no criminals, but mere victims of a momentary absent-mindedness of Mother Nature.'

Psychiatry's frameworks for understanding human mental states are inextricable from the frameworks of society. Between 1952 and the 1980s, the psychiatric textbooks went from defining homosexuality as a sociopathic personality disorder to considering it a sexual deviance along with paedophilia and necrophilia. Prior to this switch, homosexual encounters had been considered acts of 'gross indecency'; the pivot to 'deviance' and away from criminality was at the time perceived to represent a kind of progress.

One psychiatry textbook I used as a medical student declared candidly that there was no consensus among psychiatrists about the best way to understand mental illness. 'Most psychiatric conditions should not therefore be considered "diseases" since in many the aetiology is "multifactorial" and there is no demonstrable pathology,' it said. 'However, the concept of mental "illness" is useful in defining a level of subjective distress greater in severity and/or duration than occurs in normal human experience.' It also emphasised the legal aspect of psychiatry, called upon to distinguish the sane from the insane for the purpose of court decisions, and personal culpability in crime.

In every branch of human knowledge there is disagreement over methods and how we interpret data, but only in psychiatry did it seem that experts disagreed about the basic validity of the different ways to map and to navigate the subject. No other medical speciality is so influenced by questions of faith and belief: psychiatry is necessarily concerned with cultural norms. There are cultures that condone violence, aggression and hostility even within the family (the anthropologist Margaret Mead infamously described the Mundugumor of Papua New Guinea in these terms); yet others promote cooperation, kindness and compassion (Mead's example was the Arapesh tribe). There are patriarchal and matriarchal societies, nomadic and settled, agrarian and hunter-gatherer, religious and irreligious, hierarchical and communitarian. Each has its own customs and aberrations that influence what constitutes good and bad mental health.

While extremes of distress and mental illness are recognisable in any culture, much psychiatry takes place in the greyer, fuzzier edges of what's normal. As a student I read Chekhov's disturbing novella *Ward No. 6*, in which a physician gets committed to his own insanity ward and finds it impossible to convince anyone that he should be discharged. It's a story that was re-enacted for real in 1970s America, with the Rosenhan experiment: over a period of a few months eight sane individuals gained access to twelve mental hospitals by complaining of having heard words spoken in an emotionless voice ('thud', 'empty' or 'hollow'). All these pseudopatients then declared themselves free of the hallucinated noises, but found it very difficult to be believed, and be discharged. Their hospital stays ranged from 7 to 52 days (mean: 19 days). All were eventually released with a diagnosis of schizophrenia except one, who'd been admitted to an upmarket private hospital and was given the diagnosis instead of manic-depressive psychosis (a label which was then considered more desirable*). Writing fifty years ago, Rosenhan was anxious about how dangerous, and sticky, are the labels we apply to people in mental crisis: 'A psychiatric label has a life and an influence of its own' he wrote;

> Once the impression has been formed that the patient is schizophrenic, the expectation is that he will continue to be schizophrenic. When a sufficient amount of time has passed, during which the patient has done nothing bizarre, he is considered to be in remission and available for discharge. But the label endures beyond discharge, with the unconfirmed expectation that he will behave as a schizophrenic again. Such labels, conferred by mental health professionals, are as influential on the patient as they are on his relatives and friends, and it should not surprise anyone that the diagnosis acts on all of them as a self-fulfilling prophecy. Eventually, the patient himself accepts the diagnosis, with all of its surplus meanings and expectations, and behaves accordingly.

This still happens: in 2017 a homeless man in Hawaii was mistaken for someone known to be schizophrenic who was

---

* There have been doubts raised about the authenticity of the fine details of Rosenhan's account .

wanted by the police. He protested his innocence but was thought delusional; he was incarcerated in the state hospital and forced to take antipsychotic drugs for almost three years before the misidentification was realised and he was released. We know that up to 10 per cent of the population occasionally hears voices or sounds that no one else can hear, and yet as long as they continue to behave normally, and fit into society, and don't approach doctors seeking alleviation from any distress, they are not considered mad. The labels we give can summon themselves into existence; a wrong or overconfident label can poison the way people think of themselves and others.

We are today in need of more humility in how we frame geographies of the mind, and the constellations of mental illness. There have been immense improvements in the ways we approach mental distress over the centuries, but changes have not always been for the better. 'All scientific knowledge must be, at every moment, reconstructed,' wrote the French philosopher Gaston Bachelard. For a science of the mind to develop it might be necessary to discard old ideas. 'In the work of science only, one can love that which one destroys,' Bachelard went on, 'one can continue the past while denying it; one can honour one's master while contradicting him.' It's now recognised that Newton's physics is useful, but incomplete – it has been superseded. The humoral theory of illness was similarly useful, but woefully incomplete. The best thinkers know their limits: Darwin famously observed that 'the more one thinks, the more one feels the hopeless immensity of man's ignorance.' When the map no longer accords with what we find on the ground, it's no dishonour to recognise that we need a new map.

Apart from their use in research, perhaps mental health diagnoses are only useful to the extent that patients themselves find them helpful in easing their suffering. The labels we give mental health diagnoses are useful as a *starting point* for approaching and categorising the dimensions of mental suffering, but they are only ever a map, or a model, not reality – and once they've done their work they can be put aside. The writer and art critic John Berger wrote to his dear friend the physician Iona Heath, 'Maybe labels are useful early in the morning of a work – when the pile to be shifted seems as high as a little mountain – but by noon the labels should have been discarded.'

When I began to train as a general practitioner I was told that there are scores of potential frameworks on which I could learn to structure my consultations with patients. It wasn't important *which* framework I chose, but at the same time it was vital that I did choose one over all the others. I was reassured that with time, repetition, curiosity, conversation, humility and versatility, my skills would develop to the point that the framework would fall away – like the scaffolding necessary in the early stages of constructing a bridge. The skills I had learned would sink below the level of explicit consciousness into an implicit part of the mind where intuition could take over. The trouble with maps of the mind like the *DSM* and *ICD* is that they are too rigid, and have become much too blindly accepted, to allow for the dynamism and flexibility that experience and wisdom demand. Those doctors who apply their categories with unjustified certainty act like technicians rather than healers.

Leading psychiatrists too are now questioning the maps offered by the *DSM* – the Boston psychiatrist Bessel van der Kolk lamented recently that

Understanding what is 'wrong' with people currently is more a question of the mindset of the practitioner (and of what insurance companies will pay for) than of verifiable, objective facts … The Preamble to the *DSM-III*

(1980) warned explicitly that its categories were insufficiently precise to be used in forensic settings or for insurance purposes. Nonetheless it gradually became an instrument of enormous power.

The *DSM* is now explicitly used to classify insurance claims. And too many patients (and their psychiatrists) now behave as if it maps a series of discrete and verifiable mental realities – a faith in its categories that would appal its first architects. As a general practitioner I find its categories both too specific and too vague for the subtle lived realities of the majority of my patients. Claiming the labels in it for themselves can make some people feel their suffering has been validated and destigmatised, though this might be at the cost of a more dynamic and hopeful perspective on their state of mind.

Even the architect of the *DSM-IV*, Allen Frances, believes the process of imposing unjustified categories onto human experience has gone too far, and that the elaboration of its diagnostic frameworks has been regressive rather than progressive: 'The diagnostic exuberance of *DSM-5* (2013) confuses mental disorder with the everyday sadness, anxiety, grief, disappointments and stress responses that are an inescapable part of the human condition,' he said in a 2019 interview with the *Psychiatric Times*. '*DSM-5* ambitiously mislabels normal diversity and childhood immaturity as disorder, creating stigma and promoting the excess use of medications.' And he counselled caution in the use of the labels that so many are beginning to distrust, even as others are beginning to demand them. 'We need a Goldilocks just-right balance between the risks of missing patients and of mislabeling them. At the moment, mislabeling rules.' The *DSM-IV* acknowledged that much of its content was culturally specific to the USA, and in early drafts was open about its categories being products of a particular American culture.

This explicit admission was later diluted, and a discussion of the role of culture in the evolution of mental disorders was moved to an appendix, framing the manual as far more universal than its original authors intended.

Modern psychiatrists are physicians first, in that their training requires a medical degree, a deep knowledge of the mutual influence of body and mind and the ability to issue prescriptions of psychoactive medications. But their role has in it something priestly, in that it concerns questions of doubt, faith and love. The role also has something prophetic about it – because what is the art of prognosis if not prophecy? It's not so many centuries since a horoscope was an essential part of every consultation, and every physician was an astrologer seeking to understand the influence of the stars on the body and mind.

When we gaze up at the constellations they appear two-dimensional, but of course they are anything but – the central star of Orion's three-starred belt, for example, is 400 light years further away from Earth than its neighbours. If our solar system was even slightly askew from its current position, those stars wouldn't align.* Symptoms too exist in several dimensions, and while the concept of 'constellations' of symptoms can be helpful in terms of pattern recognition, when it comes to mental health problems it's too thin and inflexible to convey the depth and dynamism that characterise our shifting states of mind. 'Spectrum' gets closer, but is still overly two-dimensional, as if our conscious experiences can be positioned like a needle on a fuel gauge, or a rung on a

---

* It's also worth remembering that constellations are clustered differently by disparate cultures. For the Inuit, the three stars of Orion's belt are three hunters lost on the ice; for a Papua New Guinean I knew, the arc of its bow was a banana.

rainbow's ladder of colour. Rather than two dimensions, we exist in multiple dimensions – we each have many identities and roles, are fundamentally social beings whose minds are capable of shapeshifting and adaptation.

Perhaps the pattern of traits, experiences, sensations and memories of each individual mind is better characterised as a galaxy in all its three spatial dimensions, plus its fourth dimension of time, with every star, or factor bearing on mental experience, alive with perpetual motion. Our earth doesn't move in circles, it moves in spirals around a moving sun, and just as many traits and potentialities are brought together in the fabric of each person's experience, astronomers tell us that each star is connected to every other through the gravitational fabric of space-time. Our feelings, thoughts and memories are in motion like the stars, but unlike them, we can influence the ways they move.

4

CHEMICALS TO NETWORKS

Despite decades of effort, no one has shown
convincingly that one therapeutic method is
more effective than any other for the majority of
psychological illnesses.

Julia Frank and Jerome Frank, *Persuasion and Healing*

Even the name *Prozac* sounds space-age – *pro* for professional,
for promotion, for problem-solved, *zac* for quick, efficient,
stellar. It sounds like rocket fuel. Fluoxetine was its generic
name, a compound discovered in 1972 when a chemist called
David Wong was messing around in the lab with antihista-
mine derivatives and found one of them which seemed to
slow the re-uptake into brain cells of the neurotransmitter
serotonin. Dr George Ashcroft, a psychiatrist in Edinburgh,
had argued since the early 1960s that serotonin levels in the
brain showed a correlation with mood, and 'boosting' the
serotonin levels in this way was thought to be a viable approach
to treat depression. For bureaucratic reasons Prozac sat on the
shelf until 1987, when Eli Lilly decided to begin marketing it as
an antidepressant. The company didn't pretend it was any
more effective than the old antidepressants first developed in
the 1960s (also derived from antihistamines), but it was safer in
overdose, and less likely to make you put on weight. By 1990
there were a million prescriptions of Prozac issued every

53

month in the United States. Their reputation, and the willing-ness of doctors to prescribe them long-term, grew: between 1996 and 2006 the volume of these new antidepressants pre-scribed and consumed in the UK effectively tripled.

Psychiatrist Dr Peter Kramer coined the term 'cosmetic psycho-pharmacology' to describe the potential of these drugs to manipulate not just mood but personality, and there was a rush of hope and optimism that a new approach to tackling depression had been found. Kramer's phenomenally successful 1993 book *Listening to Prozac* spent several months on *The New York Times* bestseller list, and explicitly set out to explore whether SSRIs had the potential to 'remake the self'. George Ashcroft, who became Professor of Psychiatry in Aberdeen, had by the 1990s changed tack on the serotonin theory, questioning whether levels of the neurotransmitter were critical in low mood after all. It would be several decades before systematic reviews of the evidence would conclude that, irrespective of how effective drugs like Prozac may be at influencing mood, they don't work by manipulating the levels of serotonin in the synapses between brain cells.

By the time of the *DSM-IV* of 1994, the science behind the use of antidepressants such as Prozac was already in ques-tion, as was the certainty with which the DSM aimed to carve up human experience into discrete chunks of psychopathol-ogy. Twenty years later, with the *DSM-5*, the philosopher of science Ian Hacking summed up the wrong-headedness of the continuing project of classifying mental distress in the same way as we do other, more physical, disorders: 'The *DSM* is not a representation of the nature or reality of the varie-ties of mental illness,' he wrote. 'It is founded on a wrong appreciation of the nature of things. It remains a very useful book for other purposes. It is essential to have something like this for the bureaucratic needs of paying for treatment and assessing prevalence.' Kay Redfield Jamison, a Professor of Psychiatry at Johns Hopkins University and the author of several extraordinary, personal memoirs about mental health and illness, wrote of this *research* utility of the *DSM*: 'I strongly believe that scientific and clinical studies, in order to be pursued with accuracy and reliability, must be based on the kind of precise language and explicitly diagnostic criteria that make up the core of the *DSM*.' But its usefulness in *studies* has slid over to an unjustified acceptance that it describes reality in the *clinic*. People have mistakenly begun to treat its sketchy maps as if they *were* the territory.

Of the newly-published *DSM-5* Ian Hacking was writing in 2013 that 'for those purposes the changes effected from *DSM-IV* to *DSM-5* were not worth the prodigious labour, committee meetings, fierce and sometimes acrimonious debate involved.' 'I have no idea how much the revision cost,' he went on,

> but it is not that much help to clinicians, and the changes do not matter much to the bureaucracies. And trying to get it right, in revision after revision, perpetuates the long-standing idea that, in our present state of knowledge, the recognised varieties of mental illness should neatly sort themselves into tidy blocks, in the way that plants and animals do.

Biologists increasingly recognise that plants and animals don't sort themselves into tidy blocks either – that even the definition of 'life' or 'species' is subject to debate. The further we look into any field of knowledge, the blurrier its boundaries become. If I had one ambition for the twenty-first century, it might be that we human beings become more tolerant of uncertainty, more comfortable with paradox, more compassionate and open-hearted about the fuzzy edges of the categories we try to impose on the world.

In her book *The Truth about Drug Companies* Marcia Angell, a former editor of the prestigious *New England Journal of Medicine*, accused the big pharmaceutical companies of behaving like the Wizard of Oz. All the sound and light of publicity for psychiatric drugs was, she argued, little more than a show, but behind the curtain there were just a few flimsy studies showing little more benefit than placebo. But given how important *belief* is to the action of placebo, one counterargument is that to be effective, these drugs need all the positive publicity they can get. The sound-and-light that accompanies the prescription of psychiatric drugs actually *helps* them to work. Between 75 and 82 per cent of any benefit obtained from antidepressant drugs is believed to derive from the placebo effect. They don't diminish the suicide rate, and the positive effect of antidepressant medication once separated from its placebo effects is so weak that to eliminate any therapeutic benefit at all it is enough for a doctor to use colder body language in their consultation with the patient. We're prescribing more than ever before but mental illness rates continue to rise.

Between 2000 and 2010, the so-called 'Decade of the Brain' when the US government channelled extra resources into neuropsychiatry research, there was no change in either the suicide or the homelessness rates – both relatively objective markers of the prevalence of severe mental illness. But then if mental illness is largely social and psychological and emotional, you'd expect better welfare, community programmes and access to housing to help the most – not better access to new, expensive medications.

In 2017 Thomas Insel, director of America's National Institute of Mental Health, summed up his thirteen years at the vanguard of this global effort. 'I succeeded at getting lots of really cool papers published by cool scientists at fairly large costs – I think twenty billion dollars – [but] I don't think we moved the needle in reducing suicide, reducing hospitalisations, improving recovery for the tens of millions of people who have mental illness.' A new paradigm was needed: looking for increased or decreased levels of brain chemicals was a busted flush, old science – much better was to try to map looping circuits of connection in the brain. 'We increasingly believe that brain disorders – from schizophrenia to depression to post-traumatic stress disorder – are disorders of connectivity,' Insel wrote. Of the *DSM*, he memorably added, 'Biology never read that book.'

I asked a psychiatrist friend why one person's vulnerability to mental distress was extreme, while another seems impermeable to the most devastating events – a disparity that has been framed as the 'dandelion vs orchid' theory of personality – some people, like dandelions, thrive almost irrespective of environment, while others, like orchids, seem exquisitely sensitive. It's just life, isn't it?' he said. It's partly your genetics, partly your upbringing, and then the messy, difficult business of living with other people.'

For the novelist Henry James the mind was a theatre of simultaneous possibilities, and the purpose of consciousness was to select some of those possibilities and suppress the rest. For his psychologist brother William, 'consciousness is what you might expect in a nervous system grown too large to steer itself'; an extra sense or capacity with which the mind can play with new possibilities. For the neuroscientist John Crook, consciousness is best understood as vigilance over a 'map' of the outer world we carry within the brain, and the purpose of it is to alert us to novelty – something that might require innovative thinking. From moment to moment our brain cells stitch together a map of the world, comparing it with information from the senses and from memory – a map that is constantly being redrawn by experience. The chemistry of the brain dictates the flow of consciousness in utterly mysterious ways. We don't know how or why alcohol, drugs, hunger, thirst or fatigue have their profound effects on mental experience – but it's more complicated than through the actions of single neurotransmitters.

The brain could as easily be described as a jungle of neural connections. The most complex work of thinking seems to happen in the upper layers of the cerebral cortex: in the canopy of the brain. Branches and branchlets of brain cells, 'dendrons' and 'dendrites' flow round one another, the strength of their connections waxing and waning with use and experiences. The whole ecosystem of the brain is in motion, alive. We speak of the 'pruning' of neurons when the connections diminish, of neuronal 'sprouting' and 'budding', in recognition that the brain is a manifestation of organic nature. It can wither and flourish. In the first months of new life, this sprouting, pruning and budding happens at tremendous pace, but it can continue throughout life. Our brains remain adaptable even into old age.

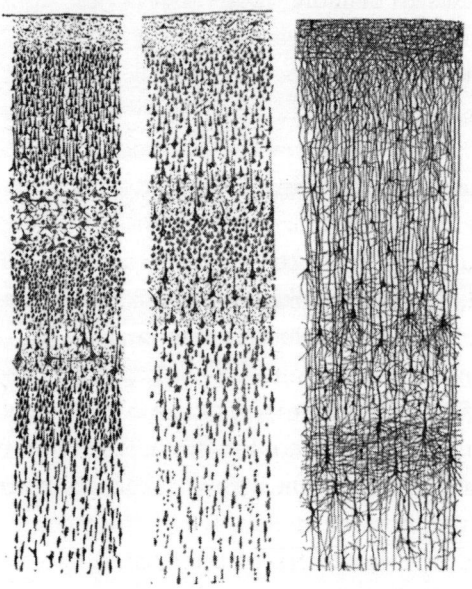

Biological psychiatry, in its strictest sense, died a while ago now; clinicians have long thought of mental illness instead as 'biopsychosocial', in that the development of mental disorders clearly has some influence from a person's biology or inheritance, some influence from their individual psychology, and some influence from the social context in which they live. If your identical twin has schizophrenia, you're more likely to develop it too – far more likely than if your non-identical twin has schizophrenia – so *genetics clearly matters*. A child who learns coping techniques and strategies of resilience before puberty is likely to manage the stresses of adulthood better than someone who didn't have the chance – so *personal psychology matters*. Someone living in a context of poverty and violence exists in a state of greater vulnerability and fear than someone living as part of a loving family with rewarding work – so *social context matters*. But despite the billions of dollars of research investment over the past fifty years, psychiatry has been unable to use its tables of diagnoses to reliably gauge individual vulnerability, or predict reliably which treatments will work best based on an individual's diagnosis.

In 2017 a Dutch psychologist called Denny Borsboom published a paper in the journal *World Psychiatry* which formalised a new theory of mental disorders that had been aired among psychologists and psychiatrists for about a decade. If mental health diagnoses have been revealed as fickle and largely unhelpful, Borsboom asked, why stick with them? Wouldn't it be better to focus exclusively on the symptoms that cause mental pain, and try to alleviate them? Science hasn't identified specific causes within the brain of the disorders listed in the psychiatry manuals, so Borsboom suggested that perhaps no such causes *can* be found. He suggested that in people who are already vulnerable, mental symptoms *cause each other*. 'For instance, if one thinks that other people can read one's mind (delusion),' he wrote, 'this may generate extreme suspicion (paranoia); this paranoia can lead one to avoid other people (social isolation), which, because one is no longer exposed to corrective actions of the social environment, may serve to sustain and exacerbate the relevant delusions.' It's a theory that builds on the idea of suffering being related to connections within the brain that can wither or flourish depending on our social worlds, not just on our chemistry.

Borsboom's version of network theory suggests that when someone falls into a state of mental distress it's because, embedded in the unique constellations of the galaxy of their mind, distressing symptoms exist in networks that mutually sustain one another. Rather than seek a single underlying cause to treat (e.g. serotonin levels in the brain), clinicians should aim to reduce outside stresses with social and psychological interventions, and weaken those connections that sustain the repeated triggering of symptoms. The fundamental departure of this approach is that it's less interested in how chains of causation between different symptoms arise, than it is in whether they can be weakened. The reinforcement or the diminution of symptoms depends partly on the connections between them, and partly on external events that set off reverberating patterns of distress. Its emphasis on circuits is similar to Insel's insistence that mental disorders can be understood as disorders of over- or under-connectivity of different networks within the brain.

If A. is vulnerable and her life is beset with triggers, a minor stressor (e.g. an abusive encounter in the street) may set off a pattern of anxiety, withdrawal, lack of sustaining social engagement, followed by depressed mood. B. on the other hand might be able to shrug off the abusive encounter, but become anxiety-stricken instead after a malicious comment about his weight, reawakening a decades-old tendency towards anorexia. Everyone carries an inner register of possible reactions that are both innate and learned, different maps of meaning that influence how they respond to the difficulties of their lives. It is the meaning *to us* of our symptoms, experiences or behaviours that determines how life unfolds in response to events and experiences – the meaning of life is *meaning*, different for each of us.

The difficulties of living with mental illness often cluster together in the way they mutually reinforce one another, e.g. insomnia with fatigue, social anxiety with social isolation, elation with risk-taking. But the root causes remain uncertain. Why, for example, do people suffer insomnia as part of anxiety, but also as part of mania? Why do people struggle with lack of concentration in both depression and ADHD? For those who hold with the network theory of mental suffering, these 'co-morbidities' are no longer an impediment to a unified theory of mental suffering, which could be explained if only we could develop better genetics, better brain scanners, better understandings of neurochemistry. They are instead 'part of the flesh and bones of psychopathology', as Borsboom put it. Mental suffering will arise whenever networks of distressing symptoms become self-reinforcing.

I've often wondered why a loss or a trauma sustained in childhood can seem to bring on bulimia in one person, generalised anxiety in another, but gambling, alcohol or sex addiction in yet another? We all find different ways of trying to fill the lacks in our lives, and childhood experiences are pivotal in terms of generating our unique vulnerabilities *and* our maps of meaning.

The materialist view of the mind is that it emerges from very special arrangements of matter – the matter of human brain cells connected in a network we call 'the brain'. But a counterargument is that consciousness might just be ubiquitous, its emergence immanent in every wave or particle. Physicists tell us that when we examine light closely enough we may see a particle or a wave, depending on the way that we choose to look; it's also true that, when we look into the brain, the way we choose to examine it will determine what we see. Trying to understand something as fleeting, insubstantial and immaterial as the mind by examining brain chemicals, or brain structures, might be like trying to learn to read by studying the chemical composition of ink and paper.

Our lives are saturated not just with impressions of our senses but with the colour and the tone of our feelings, which in their fluctuations are constantly transforming and weaving our experience of the world. Modern theories of consciousness see the brain as ceaselessly conjuring mental experience from an ever-changing flow of sensations, memories and expectations, all of which carry degrees of importance or salience which fluctuate moment to moment. Waking to a day of grief means something different to waking to a day of celebration; getting into a car means something different if you've recently had a crash. As impressions from our senses cascade through our nervous systems they are inflected and filtered by thousands of these separate, individual meanings, as well as coloured by everything we've ever learned or remembered about the world. It sometimes seems to me as if each thought or sensation could be imagined as a leaf in a stream, jostled this way or that, depending on the unique patterns of flow – rocks, twigs, deep or shallow channels, greater and lesser tributaries – that guide its path. Our prior experiences and our genetic inheritance all have a part to play in composing the riverbed our thoughts flow upon, and like the leaf we can get stuck, or unhelpfully waylaid, by the unique arrangements of our neural flow. This matters because flow is dynamic, and can be influenced for the better. If there's something we know for sure about neural connections, it's that they are capable of change, indeed they *must* change, and change every day. Given that change is in their nature, how can we make sure those changes are for the better?

It's known too that there's an element of inheritance to the shape of that riverbed of thought, as well as an element of chance, and an element of your formative childhood experiences. What if you hadn't had a crash that day? Your experience of driving would be utterly different. What if that loved one hadn't died? Grief would not have flooded your world at that vulnerable time. What if you'd faced down that bully, or got that promotion, or left that abusive partner earlier? Every choice and action has the potential to reshape our inner drama, and transform the way our brains influence the flow of consciousness. Some of the most inspirational people I've met have been those who've found ways through the traumas of their own early years to build loving families of their own.

At medical school my tutors spoke of the work of Charles Sherrington (1857–1952) in tones of hushed awe – he was the first to use the word 'synapse' to describe the connections between cells in the brain and spinal cord, and the first to appreciate the ways networks of brain cells work together in concert, communicating in circuits or loops. His characterisation of the brain as an 'enchanted loom', weaving conscious experience, shows him as a man born in the mid-nineteenth century when factory looms were among the most complex machines in existence. But even the loom was too simple a comparison – he went past it, and reached for the metaphorical stars. One famous passage of his describes the change he imagined coming over the cerebral cortex of the brain as it wakes from sleep.

The great topmost sheet of the mass, that where hardly a light had twinkled or moved, becomes now a sparkling field of rhythmic flashing points with trains of traveling sparks hurrying hither and thither. The brain is waking and with it the mind is returning. It is as if the Milky Way entered upon some cosmic dance. Swiftly the head mass becomes an enchanted loom where millions of flashing shuttles weave a dissolving pattern, always a meaningful pattern though never an abiding one; a shifting harmony of subpatterns.

Sherrington's neurophysiology was primitive by today's standards, and it didn't offer much in the way of clues to relieving mental illness. The discovery through the 1950s and 1960s that certain drugs could influence mental states gave birth to the idea that tinkering with neurotransmitters in the synapses between brain cells could cure mental distress. We're only just emerging as a society and a medical culture from the blind alley this observation took us down. Then, through the 1990s as the code of human DNA was cracked, a great hope was ignited that genetic markers for mental disorders would soon be found. Instead we've found hundreds of genes that might be partially implicated, each interacting with the other in baffling ways. In less than a century we have moved from a model of brain function as an enchanted loom to one of synaptic chemistry, to one of DNA determinism; each theory corresponding to technology of its time. But Sherrington's image of the galaxy of the mind remains as apt a metaphor as any.

The new network theories of mental illness are also a product of their time: we live in an age of AI nodes and algorithms, of information flows through circuits of varying bandwidth. But as an approach they offer some precious new avenues to explore after decades of stalemate. It is a little more holistic, allows for social and economic influences, and shifts the focus of research from a quest to define elusive 'mental diseases' to a more pragmatic focus on individual human suffering and how it emerges in the context of relationships. For me, one of its elegant features is its acknowledgement that each of us is a unique blend of strengths and vulnerabilities, experiencing cascades of different degrees of fear and happiness, elation and exhaustion, delusion and disgust, as we tumble through life, catching hold of some opportunities, squandering so many others.

5

FORMATIVE EXPERIENCES

Infant care, like doctoring, is a test of personal
reliability ... throwing toys out of the pram is an
essential developmental phase.

Donald Winnicott

On night shifts in paediatrics I was accustomed to help the
nurses feed the babies in the special care unit. I remember
one baby in particular, Claire, who had suffered a haemorrhage into her brain while being born. A newborn's brain is
supremely versatile, and often finds ways to compensate for
such an injury: no one yet knew if the girl would turn out to
have impairments, or learning disability, or whether she'd be
unaffected by the trauma. Claire was still just a seedling of
consciousness. As I held her, fed her, she seemed to hold alle-
giance to another, more dreamlike world.

The other babies in the accompanying incubators looked
the same as Claire, had the same birthdays, behaved in the same
ways, and yet once life got hold of them their lives were going
to turn out so differently. Like a beam of light through a prism
these glints of consciousness would separate into so many
colours and possibilities. From this ward they'd go out into families brimming with love or neglectful of it, fall into nourishing
or abusive relationships, find successes and disappointments,
flourish or wither under the hard rain of life's challenges.

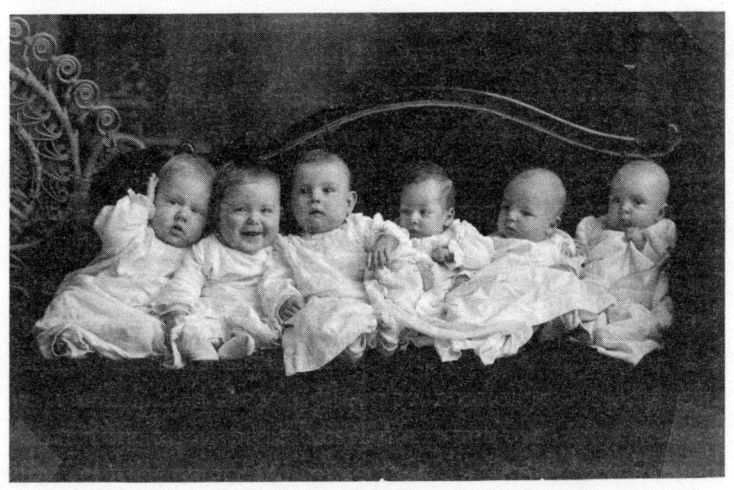

I got to know Claire's mother June a little over the weeks of my clinical attachment to the unit, and she confided in me just how frantic with anxiety she was over how her daughter's life would turn out. Thirty years later I've seen so many thousands of patients, all flowing through the many clinics where I've worked, but June's anxious, determined face remains in my memory. Thanks to her love and support, it seemed to me, Claire's life would turn out as well as it might; that June's focus would be on maximising Claire's potential and her possibilities, however she could.

One of the first lessons I had as a student in child psychiatry was unusual in that it wasn't on a ward round or lecture hall but in a small coffee room. Dr R., a neat, small man, bald with a trimmed black beard, was sitting in the coffee room as we arrived. We took our seats; there was an urn of bitter instant coffee, plastic cups. 'Help yourselves,' the man said, then, 'I want to tell you a story.'

'Recently I went on a flight,' he went on, 'and was just settling in with a glass of wine when the stewardess interrupted me. "Are you a doctor?" she asked me. "Follow me please."

'I was a bit unsettled, but thought I'd better do as I was asked: unbuckled my seat belt, folded my blanket and followed her down the aisle. It was all very unexpected. She went to the cockpit door and opened it, ushering me inside.

'"Ah, Doctor," said the pilot. "It's good to see you." The pilot rose from her chair and gestured for me to take her place. I protested, but she insisted. A horrifying number of buttons and switches surrounded me. Out of the window I could see clouds. "Take the controls," she said, guiding my hands as the co-pilot also rose from his seat.

'I looked up at the three of them – pilot, co-pilot, stewardess – in horror. What were they doing? They smiled back at me. "You'll be fine," the co-pilot said, and then they left the cockpit.'

We students were silent, wondering when we'd get onto child psychiatry.

'The adult world is complicated, hard, difficult to navigate,' Dr R. went on. 'It's full of dangers, codes and rules that as adults we take for granted, but which require many years to learn. A lot of grown-ups *never* learn comfortably how to pilot themselves through life. Imagine how it feels to be a child left in control, without training or guidance, abandoned by any reliable adult support, in a world *far* more complicated than the cockpit of a jumbo jet. Imagine what that does to your sense of trust, of love, to your sense of self-worth.' He paused to take a sip of his coffee. 'Most people love their children,' he went on, 'but not all of them do.'

The work of nurseries and early years centres, he said, was to sow the seeds of a healthy state of mind, even for those children with a shaky sense of belonging, whose homes were lacking in love, trust or safety. The scaffolding we lean on throughout life, that gives us our sense of reality and its boundaries, is built in our early childhood by the people who care for us. Those people who manage to develop robust mental health in the face of neglect are exceptional, he went on; they'd found ways of creating a structure on which to build a sense of self without help. The capacity for making and deepening relationships is one that, in ordinary circumstances, grows out of a sense of *self-worth* we inherit through being cared for by someone who thinks us *worth*while.

Children who are terrorised or bullied at home are more likely to be terrorised and bullied at school; there's a view that they may unconsciously invite threatening treatment from the people around them, because that is what they expect and find familiar. A peculiar aspect of human psychology is that we may actively seek out violence or humiliation, as preferable to abiding in dreadful anticipation of it. It's a depressing truth of human society that the most downtrodden people are often victimised and further alienated. Finding a balance between fearfulness and risk-taking keeps us safe from harm, and reminds us to be alert for danger. A child who is never afraid is mentally unwell, because being able to see threats and danger in others is to see the world more closely as it really is. And it's useful for the developing psyche to be able to see malevolence *outside* the self.

Five hundred years ago Paracelsus wrote against the idea that it is the stars that govern our fates: 'The child needs no star or planet: his mother is his planet and his star.' He knew that the constellations of a child's mind are still pliable and dynamic, only later setting into the patterns that will govern their lives. Feeling safe as a child gives you the opportunity to develop a good sense for danger. Having the insight and ability to avoid dangerous people isn't a prerequisite for good mental health, but it goes a long way to helping develop the kind of trust you need to feel at ease in your own life and mind, and gauge the right people to put your faith in.

Sigmund Freud is renowned now for his theories of infant sexuality, but as a young doctor starting out he bridged the nineteenth-century asylum doctors, staring down their microscopes at slices of brain, with the new psychiatrists of the twentieth century who were disenchanted by lack of progress in the laboratory, and turned instead to excavations of childhood experience for explanations of mental distress. Freud at first believed that much mental illness, and in particular 'hysteria', had its origins in having been sexually abused as a child. 'The ultimate cause of hysteria is always the seduction of the child by an adult,' he wrote. (Freud recalled that his teacher Jean-Marie Charcot, who developed early theories of 'hysteria', once insisted to him, *'C'est toujours la chose genitale.'**) On the examination couch Freud heard many of his female patients disclose sexual abuse by family members. He gave a public lecture on the theory early in 1896, but just over a year later (critics have pointed to his being unsettled by revelations of abuse within his own family) he repudiated the theory, and moved to an alternative perspective – that all infants are inherently sexual, and that mental distress can be traced to such concepts as the Oedipus complex, the sexual fascination of the boy for his mother.

It has taken a century for psychiatry to acknowledge that his first hunch is more likely to have been correct – that childhood sexual abuse is widespread, and so profoundly damaging to human emotional development that it may become manifest, in adulthood, in a terrifying variety of ways, not just as complex post-traumatic stress disorder but as anxiety, depression, psychosis, self-harm, eating disorders, obsessions, compulsions, a plethora of physical ailments and the gallimaufry of personality disorders. In my own practice I approach these conversations with great care, attempting a

---

* 'There's always the genital thing.'

degree of tact that can be challenging within the space of a fifteen-minute appointment.

'Tell me about your childhood' sounds like a joke, now, so associated has that question become with Freud's elaborate couch and consultation room, but there are alternatives such as, 'Did you generally feel safe when you were a child', or, 'When you were little, was there anyone you could really trust?'

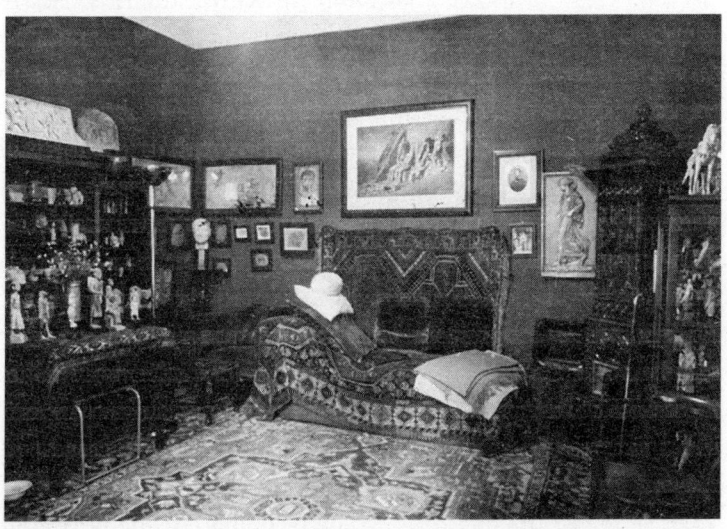

If 'heaven' is a world of freedom and ease, in which to do whatever you like, a world of opportunities, love, and contentment, then for many it exists already on earth – or its potential certainly does. And if hell is a torment of regret and restless pain, agitation and lack of sanctuary, then it too exists. In fact it is common.

The psychiatrist Bruce Perry, in the context of his work on mental distress among abused and traumatised children, summed up how wrong simplistic explanations are of the effect of childhood experiences on adult mental health:

'People are complex; families are complex; communities are complex; culture is complex. Development is complex; genetics is complex; the impact of trauma on the individual is complex; the developmental consequences of trauma and neglect are complex; the power of relationships to help protect and heal is complex.' To reduce all these interacting, shifting complexities to reductionist ideas of chemical imbalances in the brain or faulty wiring is to profoundly dishonour that complexity, and end up with the wrong maps of the mind, which focus on neurons and chemicals to the detriment of families, society and relationships.

Some animals plan for the future, and clearly have memories of the past, but the human brain seems uniquely adapted to extending itself through time. Much human thought centres on memories, learning from past experiences, drawing conclusions and abstractions from them, and imagining the future. It's the best time machine we know of, perhaps the only time machine that's possible – compact, weighing only a kilo or so, and we take it everywhere we go.

It's more than thirty years since I spent summers as a junior anatomist, but much of it remains vivid. By the end of the second summer, two years into medical school, my knowledge of the anatomy of the brain had deepened, and I had begun to learn about its physiology and biochemistry. I didn't think any subject could be more absorbing than neuroscience, so I decided to leave the medical curriculum and study for an honours degree in it.

In the department of clinical neurosciences there were lectures about blunt head trauma (when one of the neurosurgeons learned that I grew up in Fife, he told me it was the region in the UK where you were most likely to be hit on the head by a hammer). The gruelling work of neurosurgery had made most of my lecturers blasé about death – they spoke of war, school shootings, sledgehammer assaults, as if describing just another day at the office. Watching an open brain on the operating table, pink and gently pulsing, made all the neurophilosophy I'd learned seem naïve, even point-less. One consultant removed a chunk of frontal lobe the size of a plum and dropped it into a bin. Turning to me he com-mented, 'This chap likely won't even notice that it's gone – the rest of the brain will adapt.'

There were lectures about multiple sclerosis, Parkin-son's disease and bovine spongiform encephalopathy ('mad cow disease') – the national unit to investigate how this bizarre infection could pass to humans was housed in a Portakabin behind the hospital. I took a course called Molecular Neurogenetics and began to appreciate just how much the developing brain can be thwarted from reaching its full potential by the tiniest of mis-steps in the copying and recopying of DNA. There were textbooks full of these mis-steps, once called mutations but now increasingly called 'variants'. One of them, caused simply by excessive length of a particular coding gene on the X chromosome (Fragile X), could lead to learning disability and autism. No one knew why this overlong gene had such an impact on the devel-oping brain – though that impact was variable, influenced too by care and the learning environment. Another genetic disorder, Williams syndrome, was caused by a missing code on chromosome 7. It also seemed to cause mild or moder-ate learning disabilities, and was characterised by an open, friendly, compassionate and fun-loving nature, as if *joie de vivre* could be spelled out in DNA. Our genetics might seem the most deterministic part of our biology, but even here I learned that the brain has degrees of freedom – given the right social and psychological support most genetic brain dis-orders could be mitigated in their effects.

Another course looked at the way the cerebral cortex communicates in ceaseless loops with deeper, more primitive brain structures. The mathematics of that communication were baffling but elegant, and could be understood only by the strangest of mathematical equations. The cortex seemed to be where most thought happened, but it was possible to remove large chunks of it without destroying consciousness, while the cerebellum at the nape of the neck, which has 80 per cent of the brain's neurons, seemed incapable of supporting any consciousness at all, despite containing the most complicated of brain cells – the Purkinje cells.

For consciousness to be maintained, the 'primitive' foundation of the brain was absolutely necessary: there was even a tiny collection of neurons deep in the brainstem, just 20,000 or so, whose action was critical for wakefulness. These cells pump out a derivative of adrenaline which stains them blue to the naked eye – giving them the Latin name *locus coeruleus* ('blue dot'). That each of us carries a blue dot deep in the brainstem, the good functioning of which is a prerequisite for consciousness, is an unsettling revelation. Perhaps Descartes should have localised the seat of the soul there – although it seems that brainstem structures like the locus coeruleus are not where consciousness *is*, but help determine where it will be *focused*.

As a student I earned money as a participant in a series of dubious experiments: in one, I had the veins in my hand infused with chemicals while their diameter downstream was measured to within microns, to predict what impact the drug might have on the blood vessels of the brain. For another, I had to sleep with EEG electrodes glued over my scalp, so that researchers could scrutinise my brainwaves and, whenever I drifted towards sleep, subtly wake me up. Stumbling groggily from the bed the next day I'd be put through a series of reaction-time experiments, to show how sleep deprivation makes us slow and clumsy, and clouds our thinking.

At the end of the neuroscience degree I applied for and

was accepted onto a masters programme in cognitive neuro-psychology in Cambridge. To help me decide whether to take up the place I wrote to the Wolfson Centre at Great Ormond Street Hospital in London, asking if I could come to meet some of their specialists. The neuropsychologists were generous with their time: I remember a room full of academics, all scrutinising the brain scans of a child with a baffling, mercifully rare condition in which one hemisphere of the brain becomes engulfed by a conflagration of auto-immune inflammation, while the other hemisphere remains unaffected (Rasmussen's encephalitis). Throughout my visit there was much discussion of theory, and little in the way of conversation with patients.

I decided to retract my Cambridge application: the world of science reminded me of the advantages of the world of medicine, where traffic and engagement with the turbu-lence of people's lives is a daily obligation, where precision is never possible, and where imperfect knowledge is tolerated in favour of practical solutions.

My first post after neuroscience was in the humble alleyways of primary care. No more watching operations on brains; instead I sank willingly into a world where psychological complexity and the emotional dimensions of illness were acknowledged. I learned that GPs are sometimes granted the privilege of becoming honorary, extended members of the family, able to enter into the dreams and the nightmares of their patients. It was necessary as a GP to judge when to be candid and when to be circumspect, to learn ways of recog-nising certain kinds of people, ways of fostering an understanding of the background of each patient – watching them change over years, rather than over minutes and days.

Dr M's consultations were impressive, filled with kind-ness, gentleness and a kind of tranquillity – he was unafraid to let silence fill the space of the consulting room. His great compassion meant that his clinics attracted more than an average share of people who were emotionally and psychologically distraught. No matter the dark territory that was being explored in the consultation – abuse, neglect, addiction – he always found a way to bring the consultation round to something redemptive, and each patient left happier than they'd come in.

He asked me, after every patient I saw, to offer a summary of the presenting complaint, and to think about the ulterior motives each might have. He also asked me how I *felt* after each one, and spoke to me about the reality of transference – how a patient can't help but transfer their emotions into you, and that you can discern a lot about someone just by examining how they make you feel. 'And remember,' he added, 'the patient probably won't remember much of what you said, but they'll remember very well how *you made them feel*.'

It struck me that the ideal state of mind for a clinical consultation was almost meditative, getting outside oneself mentally, while remaining engaged and emotionally aware, without getting entangled (or injured, through excessive empathy). It felt like the first time in my medical career that someone had earnestly tried to show me how to be a good doctor rather than master a set of technical skills. Dr M called it being 'an effective GP' rather than 'another pill-pusher'.

Though almost every patient that I encountered had an agenda, and would benefit from emotional support, one early consultation stands out in my memory. It was a young man barely into his twenties, complaining of tightness and pains in the chest, a feeling of inability to breathe, sleeplessness, poor concentration. He was in crisis, unable to acknowledge his problems were emotional, and that there wasn't something that needed to be fixed physically. What he wanted was what any of us would want when we're in pain: a magic wand to make it all go away. Dr M decided that the best tack to involve him in his own management was to concede that the shooting pains in his chest might conceivably be coming from poor control of his asthma. So he gave him a new inhaler and a spacer, telling him to keep a diary of his breathing. But alongside the breathing diary he was to jot down thoughts about his recent gains in weight, how much exercise he was managing, how much time he spent doing things that made him feel bad, and how much time he spent doing things that made him feel good. He was to think about friendship and relationships, he was to keep a record of his feelings, and notice how his anxiety ebbed and flowed. I realised that what Dr M was asking him to do was map his feelings, and give that map an equal priority to one of his breathing difficulties.

The art critic and essayist John Berger spent time in the 1960s following a country GP, and was astonished by the range of fraught situations the average doctor confronts in a day, and recognised that much of the emotional work of medicine concerns facing up to anguish: 'the close relatives of the dying, those who are ill and want to die, the immobilized who are made desperate by a kind of claustrophobic fear of their own bodies, the insanely jealous, the lonely who try to kill themselves, the hysterics.' Berger worried about the impact on every doctor's imagination of the suffering she is confronted with daily, 'and which cannot be settled by writing prescriptions'.

To me, a junior GP just starting out, it soon became clear that many of the problems that were being brought to my door couldn't be addressed with prescriptions. Much of them concerned parenting and childhood distress. A toddler with a fever and a painful ear wouldn't come out from under the chair to be examined. 'You'll have to get him out,' his mother told me bluntly and in his hearing – 'he never does anything I say.' Another patient would call the police during arguments with her troubled teenaged daughter, and ask a constable to get on the phone and discipline her child. Meeting these lost, frightened kids, and rudderless, terrified adults who didn't know how to help their children navigate the world, I thought of the story the child psychiatrist had told me of how it feels to be left in charge to pilot a plane.

The landscape of mental health issues GPs are expected to manage without support from specialists is vast. Dr M asked me to make a list of what I wanted to get out of my training with him, and high on the list was gaining confidence in understanding more about general psychiatric problems, about child development, and the complex interactions between our biology, psychology and relationships. There were a million other things I wanted to be able to do, and Dr M looked on patiently, before asking me if I thought that I *should* be able to manage all of them. 'You don't need to be superhuman,' he said. He asked what I knew of Winnicott's idea of 'good enough' parenting. 'As a GP, you can never be a perfect doctor. What we're looking for is "good enough" doctoring.'

Clinics with Dr Q were very different, a list of referrals made and prescriptions issued – entirely without kindness. I noticed that most people went out of her room unhappier than they went in. And yet technically the 'job' was being done, while something about the manner of it was all wrong – focused on technical aspects, it had become drained of humanity, and her encounters lacked any sense of healing. A marker of the low esteem in which she held her own skills was that she seemed at a loss as to what to teach me, or what to help me get out of the session watching her clinic, and in the end just told me which drugs I mustn't prescribe, so that the costs of the practice drug budget would come in under target.

Much later, as I went through my postgraduate training as a GP, an enormous variety of subtler and far more common mental illness (and wellness) than I'd encountered in hospitals opened up before me. My education hadn't prepared me for just how ubiquitous anxiety is, or paranoia, or depression, or insomnia – often among people who are pretending to everyone else in their community that they are doing fine. Most people suffer in silence with these problems at home, with only a few of those affected attempting to see a doctor. Only a minuscule proportion of sufferers ever make it into a psychiatrist's office.

When I first moved from hospital medicine to general practice, friends training in medical specialities would ask me, 'Isn't it boring?' It would be boring if you had no interest in people, I'd reply, and were indifferent to the ways people respond to the pressures and obstacles of life. It was a great privilege to encounter so much diversity in ways of being, so many different kinds of individuals, as well as families who've found ways to make a life together, accommodating and celebrating and calibrating to one another's ceaseless transformations.

'Physician' comes from a root meaning 'nature' – our bodies and minds are part of the natural world. The movement of patients through the clinic was like that famous river of Heraclitus that you can never step into twice: always the same, yet always different. To practise medicine was to recognise that life is flux – the work of the physician was to accept that change is inevitable and influence it, to push it towards the good where possible. Humanity could be imagined as a river, and the job of medicine was to go on stepping into its stream.

At a practice in Edinburgh where I used to work we covered a secure unit for children whose behaviour was a danger to themselves or to others. These were children who had rarely had the freedom or the security to play; who had, from an early age, been obliged to navigate a world of unpredictable violence and inconstant love, and who had developed coping strategies that were profoundly antisocial. It's exhausting to live in a chaotic home where, in order to protect yourself, you have to engage in conflict, every day, with the adults and other children around you. There were teenage prostitutes and burglars, arsonists and violent offenders. It was obvious that the kids' addictions and violence were ways of responding to wounds that wouldn't heal. My own role was minimal: prescriptions for antibiotics when someone had picked up a chest infection, lotions for headlice, creams for acne. Their problems ran far deeper than anything I could grapple with in brief visits between morning and afternoon clinic. The real work was done by an impressive team of social workers and psychologists who had grown accustomed to disappointments, but who could also boast of some redemptive, destiny-altering successes.

The costs of running such centres for troubled children are vast. Despite the work of the dedicated professionals many of the children resident there would graduate from that unit into the prison system, and an adulthood of severe mental *and* physical health problems. A child that has been traumatised has a fifty-fold greater likelihood of developing asthma; girls who are sexually abused are seven times more likely as women to become victims of rape. Women who, when they were growing up, saw their mothers beaten by a violent man are far more likely to become victims themselves of domestic abuse. As a GP I began to realise just how many people who were chronically unhappy, untrusting of their bodies, with flickering, widespread bodily symptoms, had been neglected or abused as children. The Chicago economist James Heckman won a Nobel prize for showing that, no matter how much the cost of introducing schemes to provide adequate child support, welfare, day care and social work, that price is still far cheaper than doing nothing to help such children get the best start in life. His work showed in detail how every dollar spent on child support programmes and early education is returned sevenfold, in terms of the economic benefits it brings, including savings on future hospital and prison stays for traumatised kids when they become adults.

To be afraid all the time is to have a fire alarm going off in one of the most primitive parts of the brain, one which radiates over and influences the development of all the others. Children's brains are extraordinarily reactive, pliable and primed to learn from their environment, moulding themselves to its demands. And so if their environment is one of unpredictable, pervasive threat and humiliation, a self is built that is soaked with anxiety, averse to intimacy, unable to trust and which seeks sensation over satisfaction. Bruce Perry describes it this way: 'Exposing a person to chronic fear and stress is like weakening the braking power of a car while adding a more powerful engine: you're altering the safety mechanisms that keep the "machine" from going dangerously out of control.' He describes children who'd been abused or neglected in childhood, and whose distress had manifested in so many ways that they'd been given more than a dozen different *DSM* diagnoses.* The solution to all these diagnoses was a singular one: restore a sense of safety and security, and re-enact the sequence of neurodevelopment as if it had never

---

* 'Connor ... had been given, at various points, more than a dozen different neuropsychiatric diagnoses starting with autism, then ranging from pervasive developmental disorder, childhood schizophrenia, bipolar disorder, ADHD, OCD, major depression, anxiety disorder, and more.'

been interrupted. Many decades ago Donald Winnicott concluded the same: 'Here is another principle that is worth formulating: in psychiatry every abnormality is a disturbance of emotional development. In treatment, a cure is brought about by enabling the patient's emotional development to go ahead where it was held up.' Perry has shown it is possible to help the brain change the way it responds to such stress, even if only partially. Though it gets harder to retrain the brain the older we get, the first five years (and particularly the first *two months*) are crucial.

Winnicott was convinced that, no matter what abuse a child had suffered, if they were still able to play then there was hope. 'All children (even some adults) remain to a lesser or greater degree capable of regaining the belief in being understood, and in their play we can always find the gateway to the unconscious,' he wrote. Through play children are able to make sense of the turmoil of their experience, work through the pain of it and have a chance of being able to emerge from it. 'What, then, is the right way of living?' Winnicott concluded, 'Life must be lived as play.' The future of our minds, of our society, is in the hands of those who care for children.

INTERLUDE: STREAMS OF EXPERIENCE

A day will come when the bare lists of psychiatric classification seen in today's *DSM* and *ICD* will seem as overconfident as the old phrenology charts, which claimed that human faculties could be gauged by the shape of the skull as it swelled over the convexities of the brain.

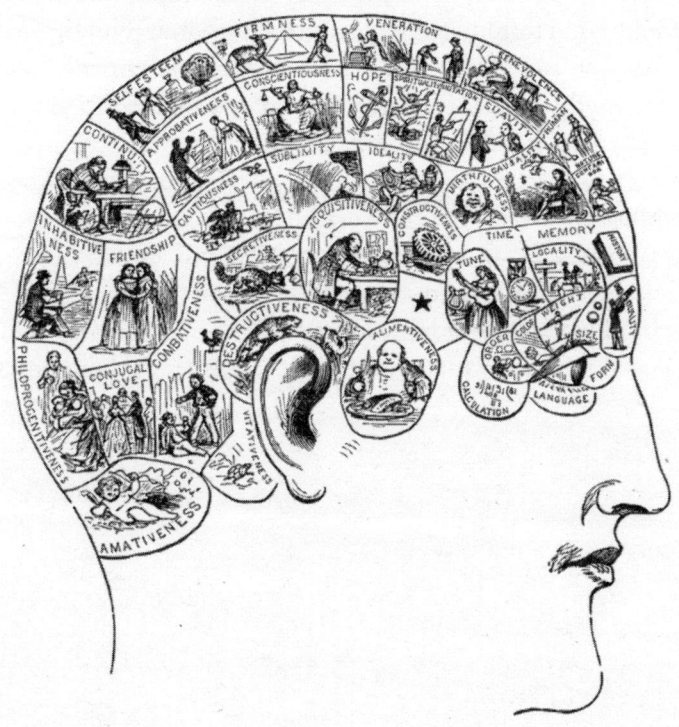

There must be numberless states of mind – perhaps as many as there are people who experience them, multiplied by the moments of their lives. In Part I I've tried to condense a couple of thousand years of thinking about approaches to understanding the mind, interweaving that story with a history of my own training in managing mental illness as a clinician. I've aimed to show the ways in which our ideas of mental health have always been in flux, and have the potential to keep improving for the better.

In Part II I'll move from laying out some maps that seek to make sense of the mind, to exploring the states of mental and emotional pain that I encounter most often in the clinic. Rather than embrace the categories in the textbooks, I hope to show some of the ways different cultures, different people and different periods have understood and responded to their difficulties in thinking, feeling and being. Though everyone's experience is unique, there are some universal, tried-and-tested methods that can help. The categories that follow are not discrete, but flow into one another in patterns that vary for each person. Some kinds of anxiety breed delusions; some manifestations of neurodiversity bring on anxiety; emotional trauma can exacerbate addiction; addictions can fuel a depression, and so on. We don't experience our mental life in chunks, but in braiding streams of experience. Your mind is a part of nature, and nature's rule is that everything flows.

PART II

STATES OF MIND

6

LIVING ON RED ALERT:
ON ANXIETY, ANGUISH AND FEAR

Our greatest agitations have ridiculous springs and causes.

Michel de Montaigne, *Of Managing the Will*

Anxious: from the Sanskrit *amhu*, or 'narrow'; in Greek *ankhone*, a 'strangling'; Latin has *angere*, 'to throttle or torment'; Old English *enge*, 'narrow, painful'. At its roots, *anxiety* has always been a symptom more of the body than the mind, in that it closes down, strangles, throttles us off from the possibility of easeful living. How someone views the relationship between mind and body influences their experience of anxiety.

For some people it is like a sickness rising up inside them; for others a feeling of horror, of headaches, insomnia, of ceaseless fret. An inability to relax, throat tight, a chest so rigid it can't breathe. Worry is constant: that you've left the oven on; that family members are in trouble. Public places can become a problem – a patient I knew couldn't stay in the gym if there was more than one person in there, couldn't get on the bus unless it was empty. 'I could no more get on that bus than I could put my hand in a meat grinder,' she said.

Fear must be the most primitive of all the emotions, and is necessary to keep us safe; anxiety has been described as 'fear spread thin'. Heightened, irrational fears are the price we pay for our magnificently social minds, which excel at second-guessing the intentions of others, but can easily slide into being overcautious, overprotective and paranoid.

Many countries have five 'threat levels' based on the likelihood of terrorist attack: *Low, Moderate, Substantial, Severe* and *Critical*. My own country has spent much of the past fifteen years at *Severe* and *Critical*, and almost never reaches as low as *Moderate*. If the UK was a person its adrenaline would be pumping, its palms sweaty, its heart racing and its reflexes primed and ready to fight or fly. And like countries, people have individual internal threat levels that slide up and down. Their sense of threat may get knocked out of calibration, like a burglar alarm that goes off at the movements of the wind, so that instead of saving *Critical* for episodes of true impending disaster, sirens sound and red alerts flash at the thought of just getting out of bed.

As human beings we have a background level of alertness based on the likelihood of being attacked, humiliated or injured. Those alert levels are constantly being assessed and broadcast across the mind and throughout the body, minute to minute, breath to breath. Any of us would feel alarmed if forced to walk through an uncleared minefield – our hearts would pound and our limbs tremble. But for some people that sensation of impending attack never leaves them. If you're fortunate enough to live in a community where there's little chance of being physically attacked or humiliated, there's always the online world: the Internet exponentially increases the opportunities for threatening interactions, even when you're alone.

Someone who is constantly frightened may seek comfort as a distraction that can become a compulsion – with food, drink, drugs or other sensual addictions. In such people leisure loses its levity, and becomes a means of coping that becomes difficult to separate from the *anhedonia*, or lack of pleasure, seen with low mood or depression. Which is one reason a mind with the tendency to ruminate over negative thoughts turns out to be prone to both anxiety *and* low mood.

Anxiety may be felt in the body, but 'worry', its colloquial cousin, is often perceived as all in the mind. The truth is that feelings of body and mind reinforce one another, and so diminishing anxious sensations in the body using techniques of breathing exercises, meditations, or even medications, can often diminish anxious feelings in the mind.

City living seems custom-built to incite a degree of anxiety: being surrounded by so many strangers, perpetual noise, potential threats, can nurture the conviction that danger is everywhere. Much mental and emotional effort is spent figuring out the intentions of those around us, drawing connections between seemingly unconnected events. 'Para' means 'outside' or 'beyond' in Greek, and 'noia' comes from *noos*: 'the mind'; paranoia was once a catch-all term for madness or insanity. But paranoid feelings too exist on a spectrum; a little bit of paranoia keeps us safe, stops us overtrusting others. Too much paranoia makes life a living hell.

There are plenty of reasons proposed for that faulty calibration. Genetics play a part in it, and the children of anxious parents are five times more likely to be anxious themselves. Being harassed, abused or persecuted as a child can play havoc with your sense of safety long into adulthood. There are after all a great many people for whom adult life really is as dangerous as walking through a minefield – those who live in prisons, or certain schools, or in communities where violence is pervasive and the justice system doesn't penetrate. For many, anxiety seethes underneath swaggering, skin-deep bravado. I've met many such anxious men over the years – often tattooed, muscled, trailed by fighting dogs, they seek to advertise themselves as tough precisely because they feel so vulnerable.

Each society has its own set of anxieties. In Japan, where the way you present yourself in public is of particular cultural importance, there is *taijin kyofusho*, which is the paralysing fear that you'll say something offensive, or be socially inappropriate. Also in Japan there is *shinkei-shitsu*, a feeling of weakness, low mood and anxiety often found among people with obsessive and introverted personality traits, who fear being among strangers. There are different manifestations of anxiety too depending on the prevailing beliefs about the body: in Korea *hwa byung*, which causes a feeling of constriction and pressure in the chest, palpitations, hot flushes, headaches, difficulty in concentration and a lump in the pit of the stomach. In Nigeria *ode-ori* is characterised by a feeling of heat in the head, or of parasites crawling around on or in your head, often associated with the fear of having been attacked by witchcraft. In South Asia a particular syndrome of somatic neurosis has been described among Muslim women, in which 'whole body pain' is the principal complaint, not low mood or anxiety, but the symptom resolves as mood improves or anxiety recedes. In Latin America *ataque de nervios* causes headache, trembling and palpitations. In south and east Asia there is a relatively common anxiety syndrome about semen loss (called *dhat* in India, *jiryan* in south-east Asia, *shukra prameha* in Sri Lanka, *shen-k'uei* in China), which arises from the belief that semen is a vital essence and that its emission through masturbation or inadvertently in the urine brings on profound weakness and debility. *Dhat, jiryan, shukra prameha* and *shen-k'uei* also reflect poorly on your morality, heightening their stigma and shame. Women may sometimes suffer the same syndrome, through what's perceived to be excessive losses of normal physiological vaginal discharge.

In Afghanistan there are a variety of ways of interpreting anxiety: *was-wasi*, which is a constant worry that leads to social isolation; *wahmi*, an unreasonable fear combined with frightening dreams; *peyran*, the sensation of being possessed by spirits; and *deltangi*, the sense that the chest is constricted and the heart squeezed through lack of space. A psychiatrist of trauma quoted a woman suffering from *deltangi*: 'The space that occupies my heart becomes smaller and I feel that someone stops my breath. I am restless and I walk back and forth. It seems that my heart vibrates and then I have a short-ness of breath and I start crying, and when it is over I feel quiet.'

There are so many ways in which anxiety can be trans-formed into other symptoms, especially in situations when admitting to anxious feelings is forbidden. Among the most common are tightness in the throat, and the conviction that something is blocking the gullet, even when scans and endo-scopic examinations prove that there is no such blockage. (I had a patient who grew up in a violent home, who told me that only once in his adult life had his throat muscles relaxed, and it was such a bizarre sensation for him that he was convinced something had gone wrong.) Another manifesta-tion of anxiety when mingled with other vulnerabilities can be what are known as functional seizures, in which there's no trace of epilepsy but the mind, quite unconsciously, absents itself in a way that from the outside looks like a convulsion. There are comparable kinds of blindness where the eyes and nerves are working normally, but some unconscious element of the mind, seeking relief, switches off the capacity to see.

Rachel had been an elite athlete, a gifted footballer whose talent was recognised and nurtured from the age of seven. In her mid-twenties when I met her, she wore tracksuits, her unwashed black hair pulled into a tight ponytail. Her forehead was furrowed as if there was something perpetually puzzling her. From the moment her talent was recognised, Rachel's life had become one of training: throughout adolescence she'd go running before school, working in the gym most evenings; her weekends were dominated by competition football and the demands of team practice. It paid off: by the end of her teens she played for her region, and there was talk of her playing for her country. She lived to play. Until one weekend a high, dirty tackle caught her on the knee, bending the joint in a way evolution never intended, and twisted her ligaments until they burst. Surgery and months of gruelling physiotherapy followed, but it became clear to Rachel that her career as a footballer was over.

So much space in her life had been ruled by football that, with the loss of it, her existence transformed utterly: life felt empty, and pointless. Anxiety had flooded into the vacuum. Shaking in her seat as she spoke, she told me that she felt nervous, anxious, on edge, *all* the time. 'My throat gets so tight I can hardly swallow,' she said; 'last week some old team-mates asked me out for a drink, but I dread their questions, and their sympathy, which is really just a kind of pity.' She had begun to struggle even to leave the house. 'How am I going to make a living?' she went on. 'The only thing I know is how to train – how to make *this'* – she flicked both hands down at her body in a disparaging gesture – 'as fast and as strong as it can be. What now?'

We spent several appointments talking through ways of reducing her anxiety. Counselling might help her come to terms with this transformation in her life. Cognitive behavioural therapy might help her see how patterns in the spirals of her frightened thoughts could be challenged – assisting her to gently push at the edges of what she found comfortable, to keep her social world from shrinking. We talked about meditation to ground herself, breathing exercises, working at her friendships, establishing new hobbies and reigniting her interests in old ones that she had almost forgotten. Finally, we discussed medication to help diminish the intensity of her suffocating anxiety. In the end she took up all of these suggestions, and more.

I saw her once or twice a month for a year. Over the course of that year her anxiety plateaued, and then slowly diminished, and it wasn't possible to say which of the many changes she implemented was the deciding influence over her recovery, or whether it might simply have been time. Her dose of medication rose and then fell away. And her social circle, after a few months of narrowing, had slowly begun to widen again. At our final consultation she came to tell me that she was going off medication altogether, in time to start a new course at college. 'What will you study?' I asked her.

'Physiotherapy', she shot back with a smile. 'I figured if I can't have a life dedicated to the improvement of my own performance' – that bodily gesture again, less disparaging or dismissive this time – 'I might as well work to improve the performance of others.'

In 1999 SmithKline Beecham, one of the Big Pharma companies, sought to spread anxiety about a new disease it called 'Social Phobia'. It launched an advertising campaign with the line, 'Imagine being allergic to people', and provided funds to put together a patient advocacy group called the Social Anxiety Disorder Coalition. A public relations firm was commissioned to deal with any media enquiries. It was a prime example of diagnostic creep: a few people who find it difficult and frightening to speak to strangers were given a medical-sounding diagnosis which had never before existed – it helped them make sense of their experience, while at the same time locking them into an expectation that they had an illness requiring treatment. Studies using lax criteria were published suggesting that social anxiety afflicted 7 per cent of men, and 9 per cent of women. A drug was then marketed as having a modest benefit in the most severely affected subset of patients. The criteria to meet the diagnosis were then broadened further, and lobbying pressures applied by the group to prescribers and decision-makers to increase awareness, so that this broadening appeared to be patient-led rather than profit-led. In a remarkably short time this new diagnosis entered the textbooks as if it had a discrete, biological reality, rather than simply the rebranding of a very common trait. A recent clickbait article on my browser promised to tell me the '6 Signs of Social Anxiety That Are Easy to Mistake for Shyness'. The campaign has succeeded: the transformation of a widespread human tendency into a pathological category seems complete.

Clinical psychologist Lucy Foulkes has this to say about diagnostic creep, and how it can make it more difficult to overcome problems.

> In the rush to destigmatise mental illness, and the confusion about what it really is, all kinds of normal negative emotions and experiences are being labelled as mental disorders – or at the very least, as problems that need to be instantly fixed. Take, for example, anxiety disorders. On Twitter recently, a professor in the States complained that many of his students were asking to be excused from giving oral presentations on the grounds of anxiety. 'Of course they should be anxious,' he tweeted, 'they're doing a presentation.' ... [But] this kind of anxiety is not the same as the clinical version, and shouldn't be treated as such. In fact, for many milder forms of anxiety, excusing students from giving the presentation would be totally unhelpful: one of the main ways in which anxiety is maintained is by avoidance.

To avoid anything that worsens your anxiety makes obvious sense – why put yourself through the ordeal? But if travelling, or gathering with others, or going down into the metro, is what makes you anxious, your life is going to end up drastically curtailed in terms of the options you allow yourself. To simply avoid all situations that might make you anxious means narrowing your horizons, at the same time as limiting your chances of recovery.

'Graded exposure' is one of the most successful methods of combating phobic anxiety: it involves, at first, just thinking about the frightening action, e.g. taking an underground train. Then you might enter a station, at street level, at a quiet time, but not go through the barriers. A next step might be to go through the barriers, down the escalator, and back up again. Each time the experience is repeated, the fear and panic will usually diminish, until after perhaps dozens of such 'exposures', someone might feel ready to get on a train at a quiet time of the day.

Repeated studies have concluded that it doesn't seem to matter which kind of therapy is used to overcome fear and anxiety, but a common factor in the success stories is time, and the will and effort to explore solutions. From mindfulness to hypnotherapy to psychodynamic psychotherapy, no one approach has been shown to work better than the others.

'Panic' is the very physical experience of a certain type of fear. Originally the word comes from the fear seeded by the deceptions of the god Pan, lord of woodlands and open fields. Pan would crack twigs in the woods, nudge branches, flit like shadow, then hide, playing havoc with the imaginations of shepherds and cowherds – as well as their animals. A herd of cattle decides suddenly and inexplicably to stampede? Pan's fault. Woke up to a thump in the night and crept from your bed, lantern in hand, to find no one there? Pan again.

In his essay on fear, the French philosopher Michel de Montaigne described panic as sent by the Gods. 'The Greeks acknowledged another kind of fear, differing from any we have spoken of yet, that surprises us without any visible cause, by an impulse from heaven, so that whole nations and whole armies have been struck with it.' There's still something irrational and emotional about panic attacks, in the way they may descend without warning, overwhelming our bodies and minds.

For psychiatrists, panic is 'an abrupt surge of intense fear or intense discomfort'; it's characterised as a feeling that reaches a peak within minutes with, according to a checklist, four or more of the following symptoms supposed to occur: a feeling of a pounding heart, sweats, shakes, flushes, chills, tingling, choking, chest pain, nausea, a feeling of unreality, and a feeling as if you're about to die. All these sensations are the dark side of the effects of adrenaline on the body. As anxiety mounts towards a full-blown panic, the body responds to the perceived threat the only way it knows how – by preparing to fight or to run. The panic response is a good one if your only goal is survival – it keeps us out of threatening situations. But panicking at the thought of buying a pint of milk? At getting on the bus? At sitting down in a restaurant? Unhelpful. If you're thrust into a panic-inducing situation it's good advice to stop for a moment, slow and centre yourself with attention to your breath, and check your own pulse. The way you breathe affects the way you think.

Panic and anxiety might run in the family through genetics *and* through learned behaviour. But however it has arisen, the way to approach panic attacks is the same. Sometimes all that is needed is to count: slowly up to three as a breath is taken in, hold for two, then exhale over another three and hold for two. And as yoga teachers and trombone players will tell you, breathing properly is something you do from the belly, not from the chest.

No one ever died of a panic attack. Though it might *feel* as if the heart might leap out from between the ribs, breathing through that feeling helps it to pass on like a bad spell of weather. It's worth appreciating too that all the terrifying sensations of panic are just the body's response to adrenaline – that in other circumstances that same reaction might be helpful, and could even save your life. It can be good too to challenge unhelpful thoughts – e.g. you *have* managed perfectly well on the bus in the past, you *did* once manage to enjoy a meal in a restaurant, you *did* use to get in a lift and emerge unscathed – and will do all these things again.

It's natural that, faced with the prospect of terror, we develop strategies of avoidance: shopping at night, taking the quietest bus route, turning down an invitation to socialise, taking the stairs. But the more those terrors are avoided, the more the circle within which we feel safe begins to constrict. We become dependent on certain kinds of unhelpful tricks, or self-spells, to get through stressful situations – I knew someone who could only go on the bus if she could sit directly behind the driver; if that seat was taken she'd let the bus go by. I knew another who'd dig his nails into his palms all the way around the shops, convinced that only through self-induced pain would he be prevented from passing out.

When the time has come to be able to tackle panic attacks, then self-spells can be seen for what they are: coping techniques which may alleviate but don't get at the root of the problem. A psychiatric nurse, someone who'd helped many people get through panic attacks, told me once that the most effective therapy in her toolkit was also the most simple: a pen and paper.

She'd get her patient to list all the situations that inspired a panic attack, and then give each a 'panic-rating' from 1 to

10, with 10 for the situations likely to induce abject terror, and 1 for those that might merely bring out a mild sweat. Her solution was so simple it seems almost absurd to spell it out: *start with the mildest situations, and keep on doing them, every day, until the effort required to get through them has halved.* Only then would she counsel moving onto the next situation on the list. Repetition brings ease, along with confidence – I've known people who've gone from managing the easiest situation on their list to the most difficult in just a matter of months.

We no longer believe that Pan haunts the woods. Our chance of being eaten by a wolf is virtually nil. Yet we're still encumbered with all this evolutionary baggage, this fight-or-flight system that gets woefully out of sync with the real risks, threats and needs in our lives. But the body knows how to live, and it knows how to survive – breathing through those episodes allows them to blow over.

In all of medicine words have power, but in psychiatry that power takes on the wings of angels or of demons; language influences the way we build the world. In the twenty-first century the English word 'paranoid' is an everyday commonplace, unsurprising. We've all joked of feeling paranoid about what our friends, neighbours, colleagues might think of us. We might feel paranoid about who's tracking us on the Internet, what our boss really thinks of our performance, what so-and-so says about us behind our back. I'm reminded of the fridge-magnet wisdom: 'Just because you're paranoid doesn't mean they're *not* out to get you.' Try adding another word, though: 'psychosis'. To a psychiatrist, psychosis is a mental disturbance in which someone has lost touch with what's verifiably real, and is having beliefs and perceptions that aren't shared by anyone else. We may all have beliefs and perceptions that no one else shares, unique to us, and so to make the diagnosis of 'paranoid psychosis' it's necessary to add an element of distress. The definition takes shape as someone has lost touch with what's verifiably real, who is distressed, and who believes they are vulnerable to the persecutions of others in a way that seems unjustified.

'What we call psychosis can also be a response to extreme stress or trauma,' writes Nathan Filer, a former psychiatric nurse. 'For many people it might best be understood as a kind of psychological adaptation, a coping strategy gone awry or a form of storytelling carried out within the mind as a response to unbearably painful life events.' The drugs to treat paranoia are in the class of 'antipsychotics' – a name which, like 'antidepressant', implies an unjustified degree of specificity. Most antipsychotic drugs block a subtype of dopamine receptors in the brain, and are used equally for other kinds of distorted beliefs and perceptions as they are for paranoia. But they don't only block off some dopamine transmission in the brain – they have effects on other types of chemical messengers, including noradrenaline, histamine, serotonin and acetylcholine. The earliest widely-used antipsychotic drug, chlorpromazine, was given the trade name Largactil because it has 'Large Actions' across many different elements of brain function – affecting not just how we think, but how we move. Most antipsychotics are sedative in their effects, and dull the wilder and more exotic aspects of our thinking – which can be enough to calm and slow the mind for a time until the paranoid convictions start to dissipate.

If your community offers no safety and you feel threatened in your own home, one of the first things many people do is self-medicate. The relief provided by alcohol and drugs is temporary – sedatives reduce anxiety but also meddle with the regulation of the brain's emotional register. If you put a highly anxious person in a brain scanner, those parts of the brain thought to deal with threatening situations are seen to be busy, though whether that's the cause, or the result, of their anxious feelings is anyone's guess.

The composer Allen Shawn wrote of how it feels to be afraid of almost everything:

> I don't like heights. I don't like being on the water. I am upset by walking across parking lots of open parks or fields where there are no buildings. I tend to avoid bridges, unless they are on a small scale. I respond poorly to stretches of vastness but do equally badly when I am closed in, as I am severely claustrophobic. When I go to a theatre, I sit on the aisle. I am petrified of tunnels, making most train travel as well as many drives difficult. I don't take subways. I avoid elevators as much as possible. I experience glassed-in spaces as toxic, and I find it very difficult to adjust to being in buildings in which the windows don't open.

Shawn recognised how irrational his fears were, and that insight can often be the first tentative step to overcoming those phobias and anxieties. He also had the humility to recognise that looking beyond the self, being distracted by activity and by the lives of others, would help him. 'The degree of my self-preoccupation is appalling,' he concluded.

Even the label 'generalised anxiety disorder' can be unhelpful, because it seems to consolidate and render unassailable what might be a temporary state of mind. Some patients I've known over the years have found great solace in joining with groups of others to seek fellowship, sharing information about helpful therapies and therapists, though it's worthwhile staying alert to whether the group is beneficial, or whether it starts to hinder recovery. The shared identity offered by such groups can be a comfort and solution, but it can also harden into something that doesn't reflect the flexibility and dynamism needed to be able to meet new challenges, or recognise that the context in which we live is always changing.

Anxiety is turbocharged by insomnia; the brain must be able to rest in order to redraw its map of which threats are worth worrying about. The drugs that aid sleep are ferociously addictive, so shouldn't be prescribed for more than a few days, but sometimes those few days of sleep can help get the self back into a gentler state of mind. Though anxieties are often unfounded, and arise from a faulty gauge as to what constitutes genuine threat, many different mental health conditions influence it. The effort necessary to disguise autism can bring on feelings of anxiety, as can living with a personality disorder which manifests as fear and distrust of others. If you've been abused or traumatised your internal threat level will be high for good reason, and that level of heightened vigilance may spill over into paralysing and irrational fears.

It was the most squalid flat yet: skirting boards thick with grime, and splatters of bacon fat, as if it had seen fights with a hot, dirty grill pan. Wear on the wallpaper at shoulder height marked out the walls as guide rails for years of blundering collisions. There was a stench of stale food, cat litter and unwashed clothes mingled with cigarette smoke. The wallpaper around the bed had been worn through to plaster, which was overlain with a penumbra of black, greasy deposits. A torn orange curtain let in a melancholy sepia light. A single light bulb hung from the ceiling like a shiny globule of fat. The curtains were probably ripped, I thought, by the dog I could hear throwing itself at the closed kitchen door. The floorboards were uncovered – not the sanded, varnished floorboards of the more prestigious postcodes but bare, spider-and-splinter-infested, and stained with track-marks of dropped food. My patient, Ash, was not in the bed, but lying along a sofa, an uncovered duvet pulled up to his chin. His shirt was grimy at the cuffs, stiff and creased with dried-in sweat. His hair was mottled black and grey, spilling from his head like cushion stuffing. He was trembling. 'He's gonna get me,' he was saying. 'He's gonna get me and it's all my fault.'

'Who's going to get you?'

'David.'

I shook my head. 'Who's that?'

'You should know – he's in the papers often enough. Look – look for yourself.' Ash pulled a phone out from beneath the duvet and held it out towards me. 'Take it.'

I took the phone from his hand. A series of messages, in cartoon-bubbled blue and white, were written down the left and right sides of the screen. It was an exchange between Ash and his daughter, in which the latter had texted, *You're not right in the head – you need to see the doctor.*

'You see,' he said, confident of his truth – 'you can see he's going to get me.'

'I don't think you've got anything to worry about. This is just messages between you and your daughter. No one else can see them.'

'I'm telling you it's out there – he can see what I sent – he'll put a bullet through this window, he'll shoot me as I lie on my sofa, I'm dead.'

Ash sat up, eyes bulging, limbs shaking, as if strapped to a railway track with a train bearing down on him. 'I'll jump off a bridge rather than have that bastard get the satisfaction of doing me in.' He folded over the edge of the duvet and smoothed it over his lap, hands trembling, waiting for me to say something.

I stood there listening to the dog whining and butting

against the kitchen door. 'I think you're getting muddled up. I think all the steroids you've been taking for your emphysema are making you paranoid.' I pointed down at the medication packets on the coffee table, beside an ashtray of old spliffs: 'I wonder whether the stuff you've been smoking has made that feeling even worse. You're seeing threats where there aren't any, you're believing you've sent out messages for anyone to see, but you haven't.'

Ash shook his head and pulled the cover up over his face.

'If you don't feel safe here, is there anywhere else you can go and stay for the night? I can give you something to calm you down, get you to see the psychiatrists within a couple of days.'

'You don't get it, do you?' He was getting angry now. 'I'm not safe here and he's gonna get me.'

I managed to get his daughter on the phone. She wasn't far away. Maybe she'd take him in for the night. And if she wouldn't, it would have to be the assessment unit of the local psychiatric hospital. I doubted whether we'd manage to get Ash to one place or the other without having to involve the police.

There are so many ways to be anxious and afraid. Agoraphobia, or 'fear of the marketplace', is one of the most common – it's not at all unusual to avoid crowds, supermarkets, and at the extreme end of the spectrum refuse to leave home. At its most severe I've had to consult with patients through the letterbox, because their overwhelming fear extends even to letting me take a step over their threshold. I had one patient who wouldn't leave her bedroom, and I had to conduct all of our conversations sitting on the staircase outside her door. All doctors quickly get familiar with the many manifestations of health anxiety – the fear that something has gone wrong with the body that only medical scans or blood tests can hope to address. The French neurologist Charcot used to call this kind of worry *le malade au petit papier* (the 'malady with the little paper'), because such patients would bring in little paper lists of all their concerns. Charcot's mockery seems to me unjustified; I'm always delighted to be presented with a list (or a spreadsheet, or a diagram), because it can cut through to the heart of a problem. Even a list of twenty problems, impossible to address in a normal medical consultation, tells me something about the scatter of a mind teeming with fears. Health anxiety has been supercharged by western medicalising culture, in that we now have so many scans and blood tests available that something somewhere will inevitably come back borderline abnormal, and our governments bombard us with ceaseless public health messaging about the importance of getting checked which, for many, serves only to amplify their fear.

Dimitri was a 42-year-old man who came to see me with chest pains, and who'd had a mild heart attack a year earlier. He told me that at home he had a baby who was constantly crying, and a wife who wouldn't stop moaning. He was large, muscular and tousle-haired, with a stout face, quick eyes and a scar across his left cheek. He looked younger than his years. 'My problem', he said, 'is not my heart, it's my wife.' He had already had one heart attack, and was anxious that he was about to have another. 'She is killing me,' he said. He needed a break and wanted me to write him an official letter authorising him to fly back to Greece and stay for a while with his mother.

After assessing him and clarifying that he wasn't having a heart attack, I went to the waiting room to call his wife. She jumped up from her seat, with eyes red from tears; her hands were trembling as she held the car seat with the sleeping baby. Agata looked to be in her mid-thirties, with floppy mousy hair, and sad, wide eyes. One hand pulled incessantly at her fringe, while the other fiddled with a packet of cigarettes. She asked if she could speak to me alone at first, without her husband present.

For half an hour she talked in a torrent: about her new marriage, their honeymoon baby, the episodes when her husband would yell at her; how she had given up her job as the manager of a corner shop; how he had chased away her friends; how he had insisted they start a café together and now she was forced to run it alone, at the same time as looking after the baby, while he stayed home and played computer games. Her parents told her she'd made a mistake in marrying him, and refused to help; male friends had been banned from the home and from the café.

'The feeling, it just comes in a rush,' she said. 'Over my whole body I start shaking and can't catch my breath. It's so physical, so sudden, and when it washes over me all I can do is find something to hold onto, grip it, and wait. My vision goes black and it's like the whole world goes away – everything except her.' She looked down at the baby sleeping peacefully in her car seat. 'What if it happens when I'm holding the baby?' Tears brimmed and began to slide unwiped across her cheeks. 'What if I'm not able to look after her?'

Time spent talking over the causes and the cures of anxiety seemed to me as valuable as any medicine I could prescribe. We talked about adrenaline, and panic attacks, and how no one ever died of one, and that she could learn techniques of breathing through them. I asked if she felt she could run her café, and look after a new baby, without the support of her husband. 'Of course,' Agata said, glancing up at me with a new steeliness in her expression. 'That would be easy.' There were options, I said to her, always options; resources and places she could turn to for help right now, today.

There's plenty that can be done to help bring anxiety down. Drink and drugs add proverbial fuel to its fire, while daily exercise helps dampen it (as if it's only by stressing the body in the *physical* realm that the *mental* can let itself relax). The author Tim Clare wrote about exercise as one of the key ways he dealt with his panic attacks, along with a better diet, medication and cold water swimming. Exercise for him was 'a great way for me to practise facing the symptoms I used to experience during a panic attack', he wrote: 'breathlessness, a tight chest and a pounding heart', adding, 'It's like exposure therapy.' Caffeine is bad, bad, bad, and you can imagine the effect of amphetamines or cocaine – they may exacerbate heightened but understandable anxiety into delusional states of frank paranoia.

Mindfulness can help still the background chatter of the mind, and teach that stressing over the future is no substitute for living in the moment. There are other kinds of courses to help understand anxiety, meet other sufferers and teach strategies to bring that threat level down a notch or two. Cognitive behavioural therapy (CBT) is helpful for some, in that it avoids ruminating on the past and gently emphasises a pragmatic attitude that divides anxieties into reasonable worries with practical solutions, and unreasonable worries that need to be challenged. It asks constantly of every worry, *Is this accurate about reality*, and *is this an appropriate reaction to my situation*? If the answer is no, it seeks to dissolve the worry with a healthy dose of reason – which isn't for everyone.

For some people none of these approaches help, and if the suffering is enduring and impactful on quality of life (and they have no history of going high or manic), it *might* be worth asking a GP to consider prescribing some medication – such as sertraline, fluoxetine, paroxetine or citalopram, at the lowest dose that helps, for the shortest time possible. It's a group of drugs recognisable as antidepressants – what are they doing in the treatment of anxiety? It seems likely that the benefit of these drugs is not necessarily that they 'correct' mood, but that by knocking the intensity of feelings down by a notch or two they offer many people some distance from the relentless, suffocating pressure of emotions. Rather than act as specific antidepressants or anti-anxiety drugs, they offer, some people find, breathing space to gather perspective away from what would otherwise be an insufferable pressure of feeling. Quite a few of my patients (but not all) have found that they induce a kind of partial, welcome, temporary numbness to their feelings.

What doesn't help in the long term are sedatives such diazepam (Valium) or alprazolam (Xanax). They provide a brief relief, but are profoundly addictive and, because they depress the nervous system, they often depress mood. Another class of drugs that can help some people are beta-blockers. They have little effect on levels of anxiety as manifest in the mind, but have an effect on the way anxiety manifests in the body. Beta-blockers prevent the effects of adrenaline: heart racing, muscles aching, mouth desiccating, bowels loosening, fingers tingling, breath catching, limbs trembling – all signs of high alert that can be dulled and tamed by dulling the effects of adrenaline. Stilling those effects means the mind can often be stilled too, as if the shaking and heart-pounding expression of anxiety feeds the feeling of it. They can be fatal if someone has asthma, are very dangerous in overdose, and there's no evidence that using them long-term is helpful. But in some people they can provide some much appreciated short-term relief.

In matters of health it's better to go to someone you can trust, rather than someone who might inadvertently add to your stress and uncertainty. Anxiety is best met by an attitude of calm serenity on the part of the therapist – no one wants assistance from someone who is skittish, angry or fretful.

The value of the therapist can be as a witness to agitation and distress, to offer recognition, understanding and appreciation of the patient's difficulties – even if they don't or can't offer any specific action. Psychoanalysts weren't wrong when they emphasised that what's most needed in the treatment of anxiety is a safe space in which to express its terror, as well as a calm, secure approach to dialling down the threat level to one more appropriate to ordinary life.

Ideally everyone should feel better walking out of the consultation room than they felt walking in, and if they don't, there might be a mismatch between them and the therapist. For the most part that's nobody's fault, but it's my impression after years of clinical practice that different kinds of people need different kinds of doctors. The best clinicians are good at gauging the right approach for the patient they're with, but time is often short, and everyone gets it wrong sometimes.

We all need a little stress and anxiety from time to time – they keep us safe and engaged with life. To step outside our safe zones every so often keeps us learning about the world, expanding our circle of interactions from what's familiar and comforting to what's challenging and new. To explore what the world has to offer is to live more fully. But if encounters with the unknown become an agony of stress, if they start to paralyse and sicken us rather than energise and inspire, we'd do well to recognise that anxiety is just another feeling, and feelings can change. It's not good for a person (or a country) to live life on permanent red-alert.

7

THE WORST ALREADY HAPPENED: ON TRAUMA AND PERSONALITY DISORDERS

They were shit parents. It happens. I survived and have done my best to fix myself. Anyway life is not about the past. It's not really about the future either. It's what we do today.

Adrian Doyle, quoted in Miranda Doyle's
A Book of Untruths

Max had worked all over the world, he told me, shearing sheep in Australia, pulling pints in New Zealand, warehousing in Canada, logging in California. But back in Scotland memories had begun to surface: the way his father would come to the room in the small council house he shared with his older brother, drunk, climb into bed with one or the other, and touch them, press upon them. How his mother was complicit, would hide in the bathroom, and be silent the morning afterwards. How his sister must have heard them through the thin wall but would never speak of it.

'As soon as he could my brother left home,' Max told me. 'He went into the Army and stayed away a long time. I don't think he came back on leave until a year or so later. Then he turned up, beat my father half to death, then left again.' This protective older brother never came back.

Max had struggled on at home for the last couple of years of adolescence before he too left on that global journey that took in Canada and California, Australia and New Zealand. A failed marriage, and lack of savings, had brought him back to Scotland in middle age. Now living just a mile from the scene of his unhappy childhood, he felt as if he'd been running for decades, but couldn't run any more. Memories of those terrorised years were thickening around him – he could hardly breathe for them. Whisky was the only thing that pushed them back.

We spoke about his feelings of shame but also of fury, his grief for an imagined childhood free of such trauma, how the experience had left him unable to trust anyone, and had ruined his marriage. I asked who he was able to trust now, anyone he could contact, or that I could contact on his behalf. I arranged for him to see a counsellor specialised in supporting survivors of sexual abuse, and arranged follow-up as often as I could manage given other demands.

Despite my encouragement, he didn't meet with the counsellor. Then one morning I came in to work to find a police note that Max had jumped from one of the city's many bridges and died. Did I have any information for the death certificate, they wanted to know? They asked if I had recorded a next of kin. But he had told me nothing.

I have had many patients with similar stories over the years, though thankfully few who have chosen such an end to their suffering. Child abuse is common, much commoner than is usually supposed. In the United States it's thought that around 1,500 children *die* every year from maltreatment and abuse; in the UK one child is killed by someone who is supposed to care for them *every week*.

In Southern California, through the late 1990s, a team of social science researchers began work on an immense 'adverse childhood experiences' (ACE) study. It is still analysing and publishing data gathered from careful interviews of 17,000 people. It asked people about their first eighteen years of life – whether they had been insulted or sworn at, slapped, grabbed or hit so that marks were left; whether anyone at least five years older had ever touched them in a sexual way; whether they saw a parent assaulted; lived with someone who had problem drug or alcohol use; if anyone at home ever attempted suicide, or went to prison; if they 'never or rarely felt loved'; if their family was not a source of strength or support; if they didn't have enough to eat sometimes, or have anyone to take them to the doctor; if they were obliged to wear dirty clothes; if their parents were ever 'too drunk or high to take care of you'.

The results were staggering. Almost one in four women interviewed had experienced sexual abuse, and one in three men had experienced physical abuse. A quarter grew up with an addict at home, and one in twenty had a family member in prison. Only a third had had no adverse childhood experiences at all, while one in five people had experienced 'three or more'. And the more ACEs you've experienced, the more likely you are to develop mental health problems in adulthood. A large meta-analysis (a study that collates the findings of many other research papers around the world) noted recently that overall a fifth of children had experienced physical abuse; over an eighth, sexual abuse; over a third, emotional abuse; and over a sixth, neglect. It turns out that the abuse and neglect of children is the single biggest preventable cause of addiction, mental illness, suicide, as well as a host of physical problems from cancer to strokes. To be at ease in your mind requires a sense of feeling rooted and safe, and if you're unable to feel safe, you'll feel *un*-ease, which is only a small step away from *dis*-ease. There's now a great deal of evidence that the way you were handled, played with, supported or neglected as a child has an immense influence over the kind of person that you will grow up to be. And mental illnesses start young – four-fifths of adults with mental health problems already met criteria for diagnosis before the age of twenty-one. Half of them met criteria already by the age of fifteen. It's known that many people who go on to develop psychosis had, in childhood or early adolescence, already had contact with psychiatric services for other problems: behavioural, emotional and psychological. In decades of clinical practice I must have seen hundreds of patients who've experienced such abuse but never disclosed it – even when, for their own reasons, they deny it when asked.

Mental health is 'biopsychosocial', and so is influenced by our biology, psychology and the social environment in which we grow up and then live. And it's increasingly recognised that traumatic experiences have vast influence over the ways our mind develops – transforming the way we socialise, the way we think, the way we ground ourselves in the world and feel at ease. Someone who grows up thinking of the world as threatening and unpredictable finds it harder to trust others, to build relationships and to find pleasure beyond the kind of brief, sensory indulgences that fuel addiction.

In recent years a mental health condition called post-traumatic stress disorder (PTSD) has come to dominate discussions around the consequences of trauma. In the *ICD* the condition is given the code '6B40', and is said to 'develop following exposure to an extremely threatening or horrific event or series of events'. Its typical features are of flashbacks of the traumatic event while awake or through nightmares (which can be in any sensory modality), avoidance of thoughts or memories reminiscent of the event, and persistent hypervigilance and startled reactions. 'The symptoms persist for at least several weeks and cause significant impairment in personal, family, social, educational, occupational or other important areas of functioning.'

The first psychiatrist to examine the effects of trauma closely, Frenchman Pierre Janet, wrote (in the 1880s) that 'the personality is a human work of art: a construction made by human beings with the means at their disposal.' The way the diagnosis of PTSD has come to dominate discussions around mental health has risked missing the many other ways that people seek help after being traumatised, sometimes mis-guidedly: e.g. with drink or drug addictions; by controlling their environment to such an extent that they'd be considered obsessive or compulsive; with panic attacks; through the kind of social difficulties that meet criteria for personality disor-der. There has been much criticism too of the western bias of the diagnosis, in that it doesn't make sense for members of communities that prioritise collective over individual experi-ences. I discussed this with a psychiatrist friend, who pointed out that the *DSM*'s blinkered, western focus is evident from it having a section for 'culture-bound syndromes'. 'The whole of the *DSM* and *ICD* should be described as "culture-bound",' he told me. 'Everything that involves the mind is cultural.'

As I write, psychiatry and psychology are coming to a new appreciation of the role of trauma in the biopsychosocial mix. Harvard and Amsterdam psychiatrists Devon Hinton and Joop de Jong have written of how astonishingly preva-lent trauma is in the communities they study, but also that expecting all trauma to lead to symptoms of PTSD makes us overlook the myriad ways that people respond to it, often with impressive creativity and resilience. They write that we shouldn't overlook 'other expressions of distress that are cul-turally more relevant, more salient and prominent, and that often play a dominant role in help-seeking pathways.' For Hinton and de Jong, to focus on PTSD as the sole expression of trauma is to 'commit an error of category truncation'.

The *ICD-10* entry for post-traumatic stress disorder con-cluded: 'Recovery can be expected in the majority of cases.

In a small proportion of cases the condition may follow a chronic course over many years, with eventual transition to an enduring personality change,' i.e. code F62.0 or 'enduring personality change after catastrophic experience' – and listed such atrocious experiences as being held in a concentration camp, tortured, held in prolonged, vulnerable captivity or being subject to overwhelming natural disaster. The latest manifestation, *ICD-11*, instead groups this issue under '6B41' or 'Complex PTSD', which 'may develop following exposure to an event or series of events of an extremely threatening or horrific nature, most commonly prolonged or repetitive events from which escape is difficult or impossible (e.g. torture, slavery, genocide campaigns, prolonged domestic violence, repeated childhood sexual or physical abuse)', and is characterised by 'severe and persistent' difficulties with regulating mood, believing oneself 'diminished, defeated or worthless', and with consequential difficulties with sustaining relationships.

There is another way these kinds of enduring personality changes enter the discussion around trauma, and that's through the concept of personality disorder. Even the diagnosis is contentious and, like all mental health labels, has no blood test, brain scan or physical test. In recent years it's become commonplace for me to consult with a patient who, years ago, was diagnosed with a personality disorder, and who has come back to ask me to rescind that diagnosis and replace it with another that more explicitly acknowledges their trauma.

The diagnosis 'personality disorder' is seen as pejorative (who would want to be told their personality is disordered?), and the word *personality* too bound up with celebrity magazines and the media. It's difficult to argue against those patients' wishes – beyond the gathering of statistics and research, psychiatric labels are only helpful to the extent that they help the patient transcend their difficulties and live happier, more flourishing lives. When they fail to do that, the onus is on the medical profession to find better ones.

For most of my career personality disorders were sub-divided into categories such as 'antisocial' (or 'sociopathic'), 'borderline' (or 'emotionally unstable'), 'narcissistic', 'avoid-ant', 'paranoid' and 'dependent', but the most recent *ICD* does away with most of these distinctions and leaves such 'traits' as optional qualifiers. The diagnosis itself seems to be slowly edging its way out of the textbooks. The concept of a personality disturbance leading to mental distress arose in the early days of psychiatry, as people in charge of asylums attempted to distinguish between disordered behaviour that was a result of insanity, and disordered behaviour that was sane, but still caused mental suffering. The term 'psycho-path' was coined in 1891, by a German psychiatrist, Julius Koch, who said of psychopathy that 'even in the bad cases the irregularities do not amount to mental disorder.' Kurt Schneider, who became famous for his categorisation of the symptoms of psychosis, wrote that personality disor-ders are 'abnormal varieties of sane psychic life'. The *ICD-10* described them as 'deeply ingrained and enduring behaviour patterns, manifesting themselves as inflexible responses to a broad range of personal and social situations', but empha-sised that they represent extremes of normal variation, appear in childhood, but often continue lifelong. The new manual says they are 'problems in functioning of aspects of the self (e.g., identity, self-worth, accuracy of self-view, self-direction), and/or interpersonal dysfunction (e.g., ability to develop and maintain close and mutually satisfy-ing relationships, ability to understand others' perspectives and to manage conflict in relationships.' They're notori-ously difficult to treat, and best practice involves extended psychotherapy, or living in a therapeutic community that, in some cases, seems to compensate for the lack of care and structure that characterised many of the patients' earliest years.

This distinction between what psychiatrists consider 'illness' and what is considered a variant on the spectrum with normality, has profound implications. In the case of offenders, a criminal with disturbed behaviour and a mental health diagnosis may be incarcerated permanently, rather than have the opportunity of serving a jail sentence and then being freed – so perpetrators would rather avoid a diagnosis. But at the same time a mental health problem may mitigate a jail sentence on the grounds of diminished responsibility. 'Many, perhaps most, contemporary British psychiatrists seem not to regard personality disorders as illnesses,' wrote Robert Kendell, a professor of psychiatry and one-time president of the Royal College of Psychiatrists.

> Certainly, it is commonplace for a diagnosis of personality disorder to be used to justify a decision not to admit someone to a psychiatric ward, or even to accept them for treatment, a practice that understandably puzzles and irritates the staff of accident and emergency departments, general practitioners and probation officers, who find themselves left to cope as best they can with extremely difficult, frustrating people without any psychiatric assistance.

'Borderline' personality disorder is the most common label – its name misleadingly and anachronistically refers to the 'borderline' between neurosis and psychosis. This category of being and feeling tends to be applied to people for whom moods shift very quickly, and emotions swing rapidly; people often feel impulsive and have intense but fragile relationships with others. There are distortions of perception and of thinking that tend towards relentlessly negative interpretations of events and of the actions of others.

The link between trauma and personality disorder has been animating the psychiatry community since at least the 1980s: in 1989 psychiatrists Bessel van der Kolk and Onno van der Hart wrote:

> There appears to be a range of adaptations to childhood trauma, or 'trauma spectrum disorders,' with multiple personality disorder at one end of the spectrum, representing an extreme adaptation to very severe chronic childhood abuse, borderline personality disorder as an intermediate adaptation, and some forms of somatoform, conversion panic, and anxiety disorders representing dissociated somatic reexperiencing of more circumscribed traumatic events.

'Somatoform' and 'somatic' are words that mean 'bodily', while the authors' use of the word 'dissociation' has its origins in Pierre Janet's word for this splitting between the self and experience: *désagrégation*.

Only a couple of times in my career have I knowingly met someone given a label of what used to be called 'multiple personality disorder' (now known as 'dissociative identity disorder' or DID), in which different personalities have emerged, and the patient seems to switch between them, with each personality seemingly ignorant of the others. It's a manifestation of the popular idea of 'split personality': in both cases the patient was a woman, and in both cases she had been sexually abused as a child by someone who was supposed to take care of her. For both those patients, one of the personalities that would emerge was a young, vulnerable, teddy-bear cuddling child, and another was streetwise, strong and assertive, as if the 'I' of the patient could move between the child she had been and the confident woman she wished to project. 'The shifts in identity seen in DID can be viewed as a more intricate manifestation of trauma-related intrusions and avoidance mechanisms, similar to those observed in post-traumatic stress disorder (PTSD),' wrote the Polish psychiatrist Monika Fidyk. Another expert review summarised how such trauma can shatter the personality.

> DID develops when a child is exposed to chaos, coercion, and most commonly, overt severe physical and/or sexual abuse, often with disorganised attachment to caregivers. The child must also have the biological capacity to disso-ciate to an extreme level, leading to multiple states that do not become integrated over time. Such self-states allow the child to compartmentalise overwhelming and conflicting feelings of betrayal, terror, love and shame.

It's difficult to imagine the depth of hurt or betrayal capable of shattering someone's personality into several distinct identities, each apparently unaware of the other's existence. But the label itself remains controversial – a psychiatrist friend with whom I discussed these cases told me that

> DID is controversial, at least in the UK. Full dissociative identity disorder is rare, and on occasions doctors might meet with persons who give the impression of having been inadvertently 'coached' by a specialist clinic with consequent elaboration of symptoms and a reinforced view of their lack of agency. On the other hand, cases of this condition do arise, and the diagnosis is preserved in *ICD-11*.

A long-gone history of trauma can make someone vul-nerable to a range of unhappy mental states, depending on their individual psychological and social terrain, to the extent that it's not always obvious as the most important causative factor. Low mood is a well-recognised consequence of a neglected and traumatic upbringing, and so a clinician might focus on low mood, diagnose depression and prescribe Prozac and CBT. The traumatised mind is more likely to be scattered and lacking in focus, and so another clinician might diagnose ADHD and try to treat with amphetamine-based medications (which can make you more anxious). Emotional dysregulation and difficulty in forming relationships, as well as impulsivity, is common, and so another clinician might diagnose a personality disorder. Swings in mood similarly can get wrongly diagnosed as bipolar illness, and a focus on flashbacks of a specific event might lead to a sole diagnosis of PTSD. But in recent years, medleys of symptoms that once would have been grouped together under 'personality disorder' are increasingly regrouped as 'complex PTSD' or cPTSD. My local trauma counselling service won't accept patients with this diagnosis, explaining that they are only resourced to manage PTSD which has its origins with a single event. Those with cPTSD are sent back to their GPs.

The author and academic Noreen Masud has written powerfully of the way that a diagnosis of cPTSD has been liberating and helpful for her in coming to terms with the consequences of her traumatic childhood. In her memoir *A Flat Place* she wrote that she doesn't think the diagnosis of cPTSD itself is what matters most – what she valued was that her trauma was acknowledged by her therapist, with care and compassion: 'cPTSD is one of the terms that my therapist has used with me, alongside others, such as "developmental trauma". I am less interested in the diagnosis, or the term, than in the particularities of the way I experience my life: its brightness and its struggles,' she wrote.

If the shorthand of cPTSD helps to make that tangible, I am happy. In general, when talking to friends, I am more likely to talk about 'the effects of the life I've had' than 'my cPTSD'. This is personal preference, because I do not experience my mental illness as something separable from me, like a pet that I carry around. I opened my eyes into it and have lived within it ever since. It is me.

Jessica was brought up in the North-east, in a home thick with violence. Her father beat her, her brothers beat her; during these beatings her mother would hide in the kitchen. 'She always told me I brought it on myself,' Jessica said. 'I should just learn to keep my mouth shut.'

'Do you have any good memories of childhood?' I asked her. 'Is there anything that you loved to do, that you could escape into?'

She paused for a moment, as if embarrassed. 'There was something,' she said, 'but it sounds stupid. I haven't done it for years.'

'Try me.'

'Ice-skating,' she said. 'I'd go every day if I could.'

In her mid-teens she'd run away from home, caught a bus to London and found a place in a squat. Her ice skates were stolen along with her other possessions. At first she begged on the streets for money, then she began to sell sex. 'No drugs, though,' she added, as if I might think less of her if she had. 'One of the guys in the squat, Mark, was nice in the beginning, he became my boyfriend.'

Mark got a job, and she quit the sex work. They moved into a flat together. Then more trouble began.

At first it was only shouting. If Mark had had a difficult day he'd take it out on Jess, yelling for trivial things – if there was no butter in the fridge, or if she had misplaced her keys. Then, in his rages, he'd slap her. She'd felt trapped, hunted

– since childhood she'd suffered chronic anxiety, but now panic would overwhelm her at unexpected moments. She'd hyperventilate and lose focus. 'I felt as if I'd die my heart was hammering so hard,' she said. Often she considered suicide, and several times took overdoses, or tried to cut open the veins of her wrists.

In her medical file there was decades-old evidence of those dismal cries for help: A&E letters detailing overdoses, or stitches she needed after cutting. Some of the letters were disparaging about Jess, dismissed her or even mocked her, and the conclusion of each letter from the hospital was a variant of: 'impulsive act, no ongoing suicidal intent. Discharged home with boyfriend.' Those pitiful entries reminded me of something Bessel van der Kolk wrote about repeated cries for help: 'If patients … are told to stop showing their unpredictably annoying parts, they are likely to become mute. They probably will continue to seek help, but after they have been silenced they will transmit their cries for help not by talking but by acting: with suicide attempts, depression and rage attacks.'

Jess got away in the end – a friend was moving to Bristol and offered her a bed in a flat there for a few weeks, just until she found somewhere of her own. It was enough: she left London without regret.

'For a few years in Bristol I still had the shakes,' she said. 'I got a job in a supermarket, stocking the shelves on night-shift.' It was quiet work, perfect for her needs: a well-lit space, hardly anyone else around, surrounded by reassuring CCTV cameras. No one could sneak up on her there. Month by month she began to gather her confidence. Her anxiety began to dwindle.

On a visit with my own kids to the local ice rink I learned that it had early-morning sensory sessions for people who would otherwise find the noise, light and crowds of the peak time sessions too overwhelming. 'Do you think you could still skate?' I asked, the next time I saw her.

'I suppose so,' she said, and promised to find out.

It's rare that I can manage to keep my clinics to time; when I was a newly qualified doctor running late carried a charge of anxiety that it has thankfully now lost. Back then I had a powerful sense of the duty I owed to all those people still in the waiting room, fidgeting with magazines, checking their watches (nowadays they'd be scrolling their phones); those people speculating what on earth that person they'd just seen go into the consulting room could have wrong that could possibly take so long. I worried they were thinking, 'That doctor is so slow, he can't be any good.' With time I've realised that although I have responsibilities to all those people in the waiting room, my primary responsibility is to the person sitting opposite me in the moment. I need to find ways of balancing both.

One day as I went back and forth between consulting room and waiting room, going as quickly as I could, while trying not to hurry each patient, I noticed a man in the corridor. He was late twenties, and was wearing a translucent tinted sun visor. His hair above the visor was oily, unwashed, but beneath the visor it bushed out in an inverted halo of dark curls. His shoulders were hunched and he was staring fixedly at the floor. It wasn't usual to wait in the corridor, but the receptionists must have found an extra chair for him.

Before I called him in, the receptionist told me she'd let him sit in the corridor as a kindness, to escape the scrutiny of the waiting room. 'He's like a bag of nerves,' she had said.

Once into the consulting room Paul lifted his visor, and his gaze, to meet me. The skin around his eyes had the leathery look of someone who has been crying long and often. 'What can I do for you?' I said.

He could barely speak. 'I don't think you can do anything,' he whispered.

His hands were shaking hard, but he managed after a couple of attempts to pull out a much-folded piece of paper, soft and worn as old cloth. He handed it over – a court summons, specifying when and where he should present himself to give evidence in a trial. He took a deep breath, held the shaking of one hand by gripping it with the other, and looking down at the paper said clearly, without stutter: 'I have to go.'

A couple of years earlier Paul had been working at the cash register in a local shop when someone pulled a gun on him. The man had made Paul empty out the till, then smashed him in the face with the butt of his gun, kicked him to the ground and bound his wrists with cable-ties. His cheek had split open, blood spraying out over the counter. 'I thought I was about to die,' Paul told me. CCTV footage had caught the whole episode, and that crumpled paper was confirmation that the police had caught the thief. Paul had been doing well getting his life back together after the trauma of the experience, but now he was going to have to relive it all over again.

Paul's panic attacks had deep roots in his childhood – home for him had never been a place of safety, but of simmering, unpredictable violence. As an adult he thought he'd left all that behind him, but the armed attack had brought those memories back. 'The worst thing has already happened,' he told me. 'Why am I getting so worked up? It's over – why can't I move on?'

Over the next few months, as the court date approached, I didn't do very much for Paul. I gave him drugs to subdue the worst of his panics – those moments when his body would shake and his words got caught in his throat. The consultation room was a place to talk things through, but he'd already found successful ways of relieving his anxiety on his own. He enjoyed swimming and using the gym at the local leisure centre, but only when it was quiet – any conflict over space in the lanes, or the use of the equipment, would bring on a panic attack. He'd set up a regular meeting with an old friend, keeping a diary of feelings to get a sense of how they waxed and waned. Through a charity we arranged trauma counselling, and Paul was lucky enough to find someone there that he trusted.

I didn't hear from him for a few months. It would be nice to say that being able to testify in court cured his anxiety, but of course life is rarely that straightforward. The next time I saw him, he pulled a letter from his pocket – it was as creased and folded as that court summons he'd shown me more than a year before. 'Read that,' he said.

It was an offer of compensation from the government for the assault he'd experienced – a standard sum, apparently, for a victim of armed assault. 'What do you think I should do?' he asked me. 'I don't want it. It's dirty money.'

Paul was still taking medication – some antidepressants, occasional sedatives, and we'd still meet from time to time to talk about ways of managing his panic attacks. A few months went by before I asked what he did with the money.

'I gave it all to beggars in the street,' he said, 'but not before I got myself a membership at a private gym, with a quiet swimming pool.'

Dissociation can refer to: the personality disorder of multiple identities, to a type of amnesia, but most commonly it's said to occur when the mind seems to dissociate or distance itself from the immediate moment. This is described as feeling like a disconnection, a detachment, or as if the world around is unreal. As a response it makes sense: if you're weak, frail and vulnerable, you can't fight back, and so the best way of getting through might be to curl up not just physically, but mentally, and separate yourself and your experience from the reality of what's happening. It's a reaction that seems to be hard-wired as an option into the most primitive parts of the brain, but is only ever meant to be temporary. If it becomes habitual then it can diminish someone's capacity to reach out and connect with reality and with others, even when there's no threat around. In some cultures dissociation is common, and even desired as a collective goal: certain charismatic Christian traditions deliberately set out to bring about dissociative states in their worshippers; Shia Islam has the holy day of Ashura in which some worshippers beat or slash at their bodies without experiencing pain; Hinduism, too, sees mass groups of pilgrims fall into healing trances of dissociation.

In an academic journal dedicated to the value of clinical hypnosis, psychiatrist Arnold Ludwig detailed just how important dissociation is for human psychology both personally and collectively. Ludwig explained that it allows

(1) the automatisation of certain behaviours
(2) efficiency and economy of effort
(3) the resolution of irreconcilable conflicts
(4) escape from the constraints of reality
(5) the isolation of catastrophic experiences
(6) the cathartic discharge of certain feelings, and
(7) the enhancement of herd sense (e.g. the submersion of the individual ego for the group identity, greater suggestibility, etc.).

Victims of an overwhelming, terrorising threat dissociate because it removes themselves mentally from a frightening situation. This has great benefits in the short term, but can become harmful precisely because those memories become separated off and disconnected from the reasoning and storytelling part of the mind, which makes sense of experience. Too painful to examine, they instead fester in the emotions, setting harmful patterns of expectation, destroying trust and sabotaging intimacy. 'Flashbacks' too are dissociative experiences, when there's a split between the lived reality and the immediate environment.

Survivors of Auschwitz and Bergen-Belsen describe a splitting of the self which was helpful in getting through the atrocity and precarity of life under such appalling conditions. One victim of ethnic cleansing atrocities, a refugee from war in the former Yugoslavia, told me, 'There's two ways of dealing with the things I've seen. You can pour concrete over them and try to forget them, or you can bring it all up to the surface and talk it through. I prefer to pour concrete.'

Everyone's experience of dissociation is different, just as everyone's response to trauma is different. During the COVID-19 pandemic I met several young students who'd begun to dissociate in everyday life: they were isolated in student accommodation, far from friends or family, and their only permitted interactions were online. Reality had been drained from life and the fabric of feeling that wove them into the moment had begun to fray. The world itself had become unreal.

The English psychiatrist Sami Timimi grew up in Iraq, and comments that Arabic doesn't have a concept of self-esteem separate from someone's relationship with others; neither does Arabic have a word for *mental* – the closest is *nafsiyah*, which means something like 'soul-self', and comes from the root of the word 'to breathe'. 'The idea of self-care, self-love is not only culturally absent,' Timimi wrote, 'but positively strange to someone whose concept of self is defined by relationships.' The words we have access to change our experience of the world.

Some languages have a rich vocabulary of how trauma is felt and carried in the body: transcultural psychiatrist Dinesh Bhugra lists a few: in Syrian Arabic *habit qalbi* means 'failing or crumbling of the heart'; *atlan ham* 'anticipated anxiety and worry'. *Halat ikti'ab* is depression combined with rumination and bodily aches. After a painful event Afghans have *jigar khun* or 'bloody liver' and *fishar* – a state of emotional pressure or agitation. It's been estimated that refugees in the UK have mental health needs around five times greater than the general population; I've consulted with many Syrian and Afghan refugees over the years, traumatised by war, and have to bear in mind the way that the culture they grew up in may see less of a distinction between mind and body than my own, and so emotional suffering might be experienced as a feeling of pain or pressure in the liver or the heart.

One study from the city of Detroit showed that of 2,000 people studied, 90 per cent had experienced an event so traumatic as to have the potential to trigger PTSD. The mean number of traumatic events the study participants had endured was 5.3 events for men, and 4.3 for women. Yet only 9 per cent suffered the constellation of symptoms that would justify the diagnosis. This is despite those criteria broadening significantly over the decades since it entered the *DSM* in 1980. The diagnosis is now common enough that I've noticed patients increasingly referring to their 'severe' PTSD symptoms, as if the everyday variety is not impressive enough to convince me of the depth of their difficulties. But I try to reassure them that the diagnosis of PTSD is severe for everyone – it has to be severe, or it isn't PTSD.

It was once believed that you could only be diagnosed with PTSD if you personally had experienced an overwhelming threat to your life, but the latest manifestation of the *DSM* recognises that similar problems may emerge among those who experience such threats by proxy: aid

workers, journalists, the police and firefighters who deal
with the aftermath of disaster. Like many other psychiatric
labels PTSD has seen a steady creep over the last few years
as thresholds to make the diagnosis have fallen lower, and
criteria have broadened. By some measures, nearly a quarter
of people could be described as suffering *elements* of PTSD;
half of all people with recurrent episodes of depression have
a 'history of trauma'.

Lynne was in her early forties, short and round with a frizz
of golden hair, a sea swimmer and a champion baker. When
she brought her two young children to the clinic I was always
struck by her calm manner, and air of quiet confidence with
them. But then one January weekend morning she'd been
driving them with two other children, friends, to a play centre when the car hit some black ice and spun out of control.
It crossed the opposite carriageway within inches of a speeding truck, narrowly missed the immoveable end of a farmer's
wall, and came to rest in a layby, unscathed though pointing
in the wrong direction.

As the truck roared past Lynne registered somewhere,
as if from a great distance, the screams of the children. 'I
couldn't move,' she told me later. 'I sat there holding the
wheel, breathing hard, unable to believe that we'd actually
survived.' The whole incident had passed within a couple of
seconds.

One definition of good mental health is that you feel at
home in your body, grounded and secure, but as the car spun
across the road a rent had opened in Lynne's world, and ever
since it had felt very different. It had become a place of pervasive threat, of restless sleep, sudden panics, flashbacks of
the accident, and an inability to take pleasure in anything.
'They could have died,' she told me, the rims of her eyes red,
her mouth tense. 'I almost killed them.' Since the accident

her breathing had become short, her chest tight, and she had convinced herself that she was developing asthma.

When I first saw her six weeks had passed since the accident. A counsellor had told her that she 'probably' had PTSD, but that it was too early to tell, and the suggestion of the diagnosis terrified her almost as much as the incident. 'It was my responsibility to keep those kids safe, and I failed,' she said. 'I can't stop hearing their screams.'

It took many months, a little medication (to help her sleep, and give her a bit of separation from the intensity of her emotions), as well as a great deal of strength on Lynne's part to get back to driving with her children in the car. When I asked her later what had most helped she said that it was time, distraction, a fair bit of sea swimming, and the *avoidance* of a diagnosis. 'I didn't want to think of myself as a person with PTSD,' she told me. 'Something terrifying happened to me, and for the best part of a year my body did everything it could to keep me safe, to stop me putting myself or any children in that situation again.' Perseverance and making herself get back behind the wheel of the car helped – at first on her own, then with her husband in the passenger seat, and only latterly with the children again. 'The accident did something to me,' she said. 'It showed me just how fragile everything is' – she waved her hand as if to take in the clinic, the neighbourhood, the city – 'but that's true of everything isn't it? We're all lucky to be alive. Maybe I'm a bit more cautious now, but a bit wiser too.'

Even the loners among us are social beings, and it's been shown that we recover from trauma in the context of nourishing, reassuring and loving relationships – either from friends or family, or from others we seek out ourselves: addiction support groups, church and mosque congregations, professional therapists. Pierre Janet spoke of an effective relationship between patient and therapist having something of charisma or magnetism about it – he called it a *rapport magnétique*.*

Most significantly, and far more important for recovery, we are grounded by the people who love us, and who we love in return. This is one reason why people like Lynne, whose trauma was experienced as an adult and was relatively impersonal in the way it bore down on her, usually find it easier to get over trauma than people like Jessica, whose trauma was perpetrated by someone she loved in her youngest years, when she was still so impressionable, and who was rendered distrustful of love and care as a consequence. Lynne was able to make sense of what happened to her, and turn it into a story that had a beginning, a middle and an end. Paul had the benefit of seeing his attacker jailed, but the world had darkened for him, become a more dangerous place. Jessica's is a longer, harder road.

Memories the mind cannot bear to hold are transformed, turned inwards and held elsewhere in the body. Survivors of such experiences have often learned to shut themselves off from their emotions, and from their sensations, and in doing so have become less grounded and at ease in their bodies, and in their minds. Trauma, violence and fear are the seed of much mental illness and, like any seeds, how they grow depends on the environment into which they fall. To begin to see how the dark onset of low mood, anxiety, OCD, ADHD, personality disorder, addiction, mood swings, even psychosis, all can be influenced by trauma isn't to say that

---

* This *rapport* could on occasion spill over into something darker and counterproductive (Janet called it 'somnambulistic passion'). Every clinician has to use their intuition to gauge when a therapeutic relationship has soured in this way, and transfer the patient to the care of a colleague. It's always a painful experience for both.

trauma is the cause of all mental illness, but to acknowledge that it's a powerful pressure that transforms human states of mind. There is no hierarchy of suffering: it's simply true that some people are overwhelmed by frightening or humiliating experiences that others are able to shrug off. Being informed and aware about the potential of trauma to scatter the mind is to begin to notice traumas everywhere in the lives of human beings.

The child psychiatrist Bruce Perry has spent thirty years working with traumatised children, and learned that people who have been neglected, abused and terrorised can find some relief through therapy, but only as a beginning. His approach attempts to reconfigure patterns of expectation in the brains and minds of traumatised people by going back to basics. We learn rhythm and body awareness as babies, through contact with our carers, and for children who never experienced that kind of physical closeness Perry has championed music therapy, dance and massage, to help people get back in touch with the most basic rhythm of life – the heartbeat – and to ground themselves again in the body, where emotion is experienced, in a way that they haven't done since birth. Perry is emphatic that the most significant healing factor in recovery from trauma is never therapy *per se*, but loving relationships. The brain, he insists, cannot be understood in isolation, but only as belonging to someone who is embedded in a web of connections. 'Rushing to "debrief" people with a new therapist or counsellor after a traumatic event is often intrusive, unwanted, and may actually be counterproductive,' Perry wrote.

Some studies, in fact, find a doubling of the odds of post-traumatic stress disorder following such 'treatment.' In some of our own work we've also found that the most effective interventions involve educating and supporting the existing social support network, particularly the family, about the known and predictable effects of acute trauma and offering access to more therapeutic support if – and only if – the family sees extreme or prolonged post-traumatic symptoms.

Symptoms of dissociation and rushing adrenaline that characterise PTSD often began with good reason: as a response to a traumatic event they often had excellent survival value. But when it endures beyond its usefulness it has become damaging and futile. Perry and his team cared for the children who survived the massacre at Waco, when all but a few followers of a messianic cult leader called David Koresh were killed. 'The children who did best after the Davidian apocalypse', Perry wrote, 'were the ones who were released afterwards into the healthiest and most loving worlds, whether it was with family who still believed in the Davidian ways or with loved ones who rejected Koresh entirely.' Everyone's trauma and their response to it is unique, but to be given the opportunity to care, and be cared for, is the best way to get back at ease with your mind and body.

For people who knew no safety as children, that time cannot be lived again. But a sense of safety, grounding and ease *can* be restored. Some people are frightened that the emotional damage they sustained is irrevocable, but our bodies and minds are part of nature, and nature has a genius for compensation, adaptation, regrowth and rebirth. The therapist Clarissa Pinkola Estés describes adaptation to insufferable traumatic memories as a kind of 'conscious forgetting', suggesting that it's possible, with support, to deliberately distance oneself from such a history and make a conscious decision to lose sight of traumatic history, 'thereby living in a new landscape, creating new life and new experiences to think about instead of the old ones. This kind of forgetting does not erase memory, it lays the motion surrounding the memory to rest.'

One of the last times I saw Paul, he pulled a plant pot from a supermarket bag. Coming up out of its soil was a dead, woody stump, but from halfway up the stem a flower had erupted. 'Look at this!' he said. 'I thought it was incredible, I had to bring it to show you. That flower! I was so sure it was dead.'

8

A FIRE HOSE OF EPIPHANIES: ON MANIA AND ELATION, WONDER AND AWE

> It seemed as though the refreshing breath of some
> kind goddess of wisdom were being gently blown
> against the surface of my brain ... So delicate, so
> crisp and exhilarating was it that words fail me in my
> attempt to describe it.
>
> Clifford Beers, *A Mind That Found Itself*

The last time I saw one of the doctors at your place ... it wasn't very good. He wasn't very good. So I've been nervous about calling.

I'm sorry to hear that. What would you like to talk about?

I'm nervous most of the time, and feel low, feel down, but then the next minute I feel high, on edge, can't sleep, lose my rag. My friend says I'm bipolar.

What do you mean by bipolar?

You know, manic-depressive. She says she looked it up, and it sounds just like me. She said, 'Hayley, you're bipolar, that's your problem.' Do you think that's possible?

Well, we could start by having a conversation about you, and what's been going on with you. Tell me about your life.

Well. I'm living in this ... wait, no, I'll start with my job

– I have this temporary job, and the rest of the crew there, they're not very understanding.

Understanding?

They are kind of brutal, harsh jokes and macho stuff all the time. Make fun of me for being the only girl. But anyway, I'm not going to be in that job much longer.

Who is it for?

The council. But I hate that job, I'm moving on.

Where are you living?

Just a temporary place – a friend of a friend let it to me but they're coming back so I have to move out.

When will that happen?

End of this month.

That sounds difficult.

That's part of it.

[*Pause.*]

What else is going on?

Well, I've got a new job starting next month, so I need to start looking over there for somewhere to stay. A nice job, for a housing charity. Good people.

Where?

Glasgow.

So you've got to find somewhere to live in Glasgow?

Mm. That's probably part of maybe why I'm so up and down. I've got a couple of old pals there, I could start with them, sofa-surf, maybe.

Not easy, having to change job *and* where you live at the same time.

For a while now, two years, I've been seeing a therapist, and she says that I should try medication. But if I'm bipolar, do they have medication for that?

Yes, but it's not for everyone. Tell me why your therapist thinks you're bipolar.

Can you tell me about the medications first?

People who are bipolar, or manic-depressive, they often have these slow, long swings between feeling really down or depressed, can hardly get out bed, can't work, feeling that they can't get any pleasure out of anything, nothing is enjoyable, even that life isn't worth living. And I'd be curious to know whether you've had periods like that.

Hmm.

And then for someone who is bipolar, after months or years, they might have these other periods when they feel really high, or agitated, and can hardly sleep. They might feel like they can do anything, they're disinhibited, talk *at* people rather than *with* people, tell people what they really think of them, run up big bills on their credit card, take on too many projects, are convinced that everything they do is going to be a great success. Which sometimes doesn't cause too much in the way of problems, but sometimes it really can.

What problems?

The police get involved because they are behaving in a way dangerous to themselves or to others.

Like what?

I've known people try to walk along the edge of a high bridge because they believe they're invincible, or immortal. Or they spend all the family's savings because they're convinced their latest moneymaking scheme is going to make them a millionaire. They get caught for fraud by the police, or get brought in when they believe they can fly. I had a patient once who'd unscrew all the doors of her house because they 'blocked energy' – including the front door. Those are the kind of behaviours that might make me think someone has a tendency towards the *manic* part of manic-depressive – the old name for bipolar.

And the medication?

There's good evidence that if you're bipolar, it helps to be on lithium as a regular medication – it can even out the swings. But people who've a tendency to go high, even when they are feeling low, they should avoid antidepressants, because antidepressants can trigger them to go high.

So if you're not like that, not as extreme, you're just having a mood that goes up and down, then you're not bipolar?

Well there are different levels of it, but we all have ups and downs in mood, and some people's are just more extreme, because of their nature but also because of their circumstances. But if the swings are milder then I wouldn't necessarily call that bipolar. Some psychiatrists divide bipolar into type 1 and 2, with 2 being milder. But other psychiatrists say there are as many types of bipolar as there are people with mood swings. So there are different views out there. The mild end of it gets called 'cyclothymic' – thymic means mood – to get across the idea of cycling swings of mood. But that doesn't usually need medications like lithium.

It's exhausting, having to live like that, up and down all the time. Do they have drugs for it if you're more mildly affected?

I'm quite happy to talk about what's been going on with you.

No, just go on about the medication.

For people whose mood goes up and down in cycles, but they're never so depressed that they're suicidal, and never so high that they get frankly delusional or dangerous, or get into trouble with the police, there are some medications that can help even out the swings. Some people still get periods when they feel high, they're full of energy, start loads of projects, don't sleep very well, their minds filling up with ideas, but it can be mingled with a bad feeling too, of being on edge and unsettled and irritable with everyone and everything. Some of those people appreciate taking mood stabilisers, which are actually anti-epilepsy medicines, but even in people without epilepsy, they seem to help keep

the mood more stable. Things like carbamazepine or lam-
otrigine; they can slow down those swings in mood, or at
least keep the swings or cycles from going too low or too
high.

I'm sort of low, I mean sad, most of the time. Most of the
time I'm sad. And I don't know why. On the face of it my life
looks good – things are good, I've got a great new job, I'm
moving to somewhere I have friends, I feel as if there's no
reason I should be – sad.

When was the last time you'd say you felt really well?
How about your teens – were you happy in your teens?

Oh, my teens, no, they were a nightmare. I actually moved
out when I was about fourteen, I moved out to live with my
aunt, who had a spare room. She was kind, but working all
the time. She left me to myself. And then at 17 something
terrible happened, at a party. I was drunk, there was this boy.
Afterwards I tried telling the police, but they said I shouldn't
get drunk – you know, someone there actually told me that I
was asking for it, getting drunk, losing control. Someone said
that to me, as if it was my fault.

I'm sorry to hear that. [*Pause.*] And when you were a
child, at primary school, did you have times when you were
you happy?

God no.

Maybe there *are* some reasons why you feel sad. It doesn't
sound like for much of your early years you felt safe or that
there were people around you that you trusted. I quite often
meet people who feel sad about the childhood they *didn't*
get. A kind of grief for the way things turned out.

But I'm fine now, managing. I have no reason to feel low.
It doesn't make sense.

But you told me you *do* feel low, and sometimes high –
that's the truth of your feelings. Some people have moods
that go up and down because they didn't learn well how

to manage their feelings when they were small. It's hard to learn to manage your emotions as a child when you never feel safe, or you don't have people around you who you trust.

Why has no one spoken to me about this before? Why have none of the doctors asked me about this stuff?

It's easier face to face. If you can come into the surgery we can meet properly – it's not easy on the phone.

Yes but the phone suits me, if you don't mind. You were saying about the medications.

There's another kind of medication we use sometimes when insomnia and agitation are the main problem, when people feel strung out and can't rest, but they feel low at the same time as feeling hyped up, on edge. There's one called mirtazapine, one called trazodone. And they're antidepressants of sorts, but they're sedating, can help you to sleep, and make you feel a bit calmer. Some people prefer these to the usual antidepressants, like fluoxetine and sertraline, because those ones can make you feel more uptight at least for the first few weeks, and don't particularly help your sleep, and they can affect your libido. So some people prefer to go for mirtazapine or trazodone.

And if you're really bipolar? Can you use them?

I wouldn't, no, because they're still antidepressants, so there's a small chance they can make you go high. But most of the people I see who feel uptight and agitated and on edge aren't truly bipolar. It's more like what we were just discussing, that they can't rely on or keep a handle on their own emotions. If your home wasn't a restful place growing up, and you were never able to relax, or feel at home in your own body, then you can end up with difficulties keeping your emotions under control. Rather than being truly bipolar those people often feel a bit low much of the time, but every so often they break out of it into a period of what can look a bit like mania, but it's not real mania, it's just a kind of overflow of agitation from someone who had to learn to repress too much in the past. Rather than being manic, it's like a burst of static, or boiling over, a load of fizzing energy coming out after being too long held under. They're not bipolar, but they do have difficulties in managing their feelings. I might say that they're having difficulty learning as an adult the kind of regulation of their state of mind that other people learned when they were small.

[*Small voice*] And is there nothing you can give that helps people get through that?

In extreme cases the psychiatrists recommend strong kinds of sedatives, things like olanzapine and quetiapine, that can blunt the sharpness of the agitation. But those medications can slow you down and make you put on weight. And the slightly sedating antidepressant drugs occasionally help too, mirtazapine and trazodone. Another alternative for some is taking beta-blockers to block the effects of adrenaline in their body, if they aren't asthmatic. Sometimes that's all that people need, when they're feeling overwhelmed and shaky with palpitations in their heart, and sweaty palms – blocking the adrenaline stops those kinds of manifestations of stress, and that's enough to make them feel a bit better, so that they can think straight and focus on other ways of getting calm.

But they don't affect your mind? Just your heart and your sweat? That doesn't sound worth it.

It's a funny thing about the mind, but changing how you feel in your body is half the battle.

They're not addictive, are they?

Not really, you can just take them when you need them, and then stop, and it's better to only use them short term. I know a fair few people who only use them sometimes – when they've got a lot on or a stressful meeting or when they have to go out and do something difficult. For them it's somewhere to start, and gives them a bit of agency while they are learning other ways to get their feelings and emotions under control.

I wouldn't mind trying something like that.

Would you come in and see me?

When?

Today? Next week? It would be good to make a start.

The first time I met him Will looked like an escapee from Victorian England, with mutton-chop sideburns, whiskers and a suit of Harris tweed. From time to time he'd pull a watch from his pocket, flip it open and grunt. His accent was brassy, polished to a fine cutting edge; occasionally he'd let a vowel slip and I'd wonder at its authenticity. 'I say, really, I can't sit around all day, and you must be getting on,' he'd say. 'I don't need a doctor, I don't know why I'm even here. My brother made the appointment.'

'He told me he was worried about you. He mentioned that you hadn't been sleeping well.'

'I don't need to sleep. I'm fine. I've just been busy.'

'Busy?'

'I can't tell you at what. It's very important, top secret, my finest work ever. I'm in correspondence with the Pope and the Queen. Any day now I'll have to leave for London and Rome.'

His educational history was, he reported, exemplary: an impressive roll-call of prestigious institutions and esoteric disciplines, all completed with honours and followed by offers of lucrative and world-transforming work. I looked at his address – a large, light-filled flat in one of Edinburgh's leafier streets – not too far from his brother's house, so that he could be kept under a watchful eye.

Consultations with Will were never boring – he was fun and energetic to be around. 'Tell you what, Dr Francis, I don't reckon I could do your job, listening to people's problems all day – not me. Moan moan moan; I'd wouldn't be able to help myself. I'd tell them all to get a life, pull themselves together.' The wax on his moustache glistened; he finessed it to a point. 'Life is just too short to spend it listening to other people's problems.'

Will's prescription of lithium had been going for a few years now. I'd seen his records, and could guess how things had been for him in the years before it was prescribed. The time the police dragged him down off some cliffs when he thought he could fly. The time he was pulled over for speeding while test driving a Lamborghini. The time he'd walked to the English border, night and day, because he was sure some epiphany was waiting for him there. 'I just didn't need to sleep,' he said, when I asked him about it.

'And what was your epiphany?' I asked. He laughed.

'There wasn't one! I just turned round and walked back again.'

Then there were the lows. Weeks when he wouldn't leave the house, would neglect to get dressed, would shuffle from his room to the kitchen and back again like a melancholic ghost. Ghastly encounters with emptiness of all feeling, except a sense of futility. But as far as his brother was concerned, they were still to be preferred to the highs.

Imagine having a hidden switch that could flick on only the best aspects of going high: its pressing airlift of ideas, its soaring, thrilling sense of being more truly alive, its sensation of careering through life fuelled by brilliant energies that by turns provoke and inspire. Power! Leadership! Understanding! All the creaking cogs that slow life down have been loosened and lubricated; inconveniences and obstructions dissolve or are blasted away. Ecstatic glories of ideas tumble effortlessly from the mind and into half-begun plans and actions. Sleep feels like wasted time, optional for people gifted with such heightened sensibility. Everyone you encounter seems more fascinating, thrilling, sexier, their conversation more rewarding. Who wouldn't want to live in such a state of mind?

It's just as well we have centuries-worth of myths and stories that warn otherwise: the poisoned chalice, the enchanted apple, the Midas touch, Icarus who flew too close to the sun. No one has such a switch, but if they did, then the temptation would be strong to tape it to 'off' and mark it DO NOT TOUCH. I've never met someone prone to elation and mania that hasn't experienced its dark side, and been frightened by its insomnia, lack of concentration, pressured urgency, the frustration that builds with the decrepitude of everyone else in the slow, boring world.

Leonard Woolf wrote of his wife Virginia's episodes of elation followed by desolation.

> Four times in her life the symptoms would not go and she passed across the border which divides what we call insanity from sanity … there were two distinct stages which are technically called manic-depressive. In the manic stage she was extremely excited; the mind raced; she talked volubly and, at the height of the attack, incoherently … During the depressive stage all her thoughts and emotions were the exact opposite of what they had been in the manic stage. She was in the depths of melancholia and despair; she scarcely spoke; refused to eat; refused to believe that she was ill and insisted that her condition was due to her own guilt; at the height of this stage she tried to commit suicide, in the 1895 attack, by jumping out of a window, in 1915 by taking an overdose of Veronal; in 1941 she drowned herself in the river Ouse … There were moments or periods during

her illness, particularly in the excited stage, when she was what could be called 'raving mad' and her thoughts and speech became completely uncoordinated, and she had no contact with reality. Except for these periods, she remained all through her illness, even when most insane, terribly sane in three-quarters of her mind.

The earliest nineteenth-century psychiatrists called manic depression 'circular insanity' or 'insanity of double form', because every manic episode seemed to trigger its own undoing, to sow the seeds of its own dark flowering of depression. Those depressions sap strength from life, wring will and energy from the body, disturb sleep and render ugly everything that previously felt so gloriously beautiful. It can be quite soon after a high has peaked and is on its way down that energy cedes to an exhausting restlessness. Where there was clarity a fog of regret descends, along with a jaded, washed-out misery. All deep depressions feel black and hopeless, but the misery of bipolar depressions is often worsened by the consequences of the manic mêlée that preceded it. Sometimes both feelings, high and low, arrive at once; these 'mixed states' are feared and dreaded by sufferers. To feel agitated despair, and at the same time be restless with half-started plans and weeks of minimal sleep, is to experience a special kind of hell. Sleep is utterly fundamental to our well-being – and total insomnia fatal within a week or so. We are dynamic beings who must move between periods of rest and wakefulness, between moods high and low. But virtue and ease lie in the balance between extremes – are never an extreme in themselves.

It's exhausting to spend a life trekking from the depths of human feeling to the peaks and back again; for some people as often as every few weeks. But there's hope, too: in the past fifty years it's been confirmed ever more forcefully that, when it comes to manic depression or bipolar illness, medication helps. Therapy helps too, especially when it comes to understanding and recognising the triggers that start those flights of elevated mood.

The most effective psychiatric drug for severe bipolar illness is the simplest: lithium carbonate, an elemental salt. Study after study has shown how effectively it dampens swings in mood. But to work properly the dose of lithium has to be closely controlled. 'All things are poison, and nothing is without poison,' wrote Paracelsus 500 years ago; 'the dosage alone makes it so a thing is not a poison.' And all of my patients who take lithium have their blood levels tested regularly or risk kidney and thyroid damage.

Lithium's origin story as a drug is one of strange serendipity: in the 1940s an Australian researcher, John Cade, was trying to figure out whether there might be a chemical that *caused* mania. He collected the urine of people experiencing it, and injected it into guinea pigs. The undissolved salts in the urine seemed to provoke fatal convulsions, and so to resolve the problem he added lithium, solely to help those salts dissolve. When the guinea pigs were given the lithium-enriched urine they became more docile, gentle and relaxed. To establish a safe dose Cade began to take lithium himself, before trying it out on ten of his manic patients, as well as six of his psychotic patients and six of those who were depressed. Only the manic patients showed an improvement, and that improvement was dramatic.

The use of lithium to calm the mind already had a human history: in the nineteenth century the labels on Perrier and Vichy mineral waters boasted their lithium content, because of a perception of it being good for 'nerves'. It was thought to dissolve 'brain gout', as well as kidney and bladder stones. The soft drink 7Up included added lithium until 1950, again promoted for its effects on mood. There have been studies that have found a tentative link between high lithium levels in tap water and reduced community suicide rates. No one knows how this works: brain cells communicate through minuscule pores of sodium, potassium and calcium, and lithium must effect a multiplicity of changes across those vital channels of the brain.

It wasn't until five years after Cade's Australian study that his research on lithium was followed up, by Mogens Schou in Denmark, and the drug was offered as a treatment for manic episodes as a kind of sedative. When Schou's study concluded, his patients' supply of lithium was curtailed; it was later discovered several had found it so helpful that they went on to source raw lithium themselves. As an elemental salt it can never be patented, which is perhaps why it took so long to catch on in the world of pharmaceutical psychiatry (which depends on patentable drugs to recoup costs and reward shareholders).

It's not without side effects – dizziness, thirst, vomiting, blurred vision – but within certain strict dosing schedules there's no other drug that has done so much to even out the intensity of both manic highs and debilitating lows.

Back to that imaginary switch that could offer the high flights of ideas that characterise mania: maybe if it was possible to have a dialled-down version of such a switch, one that energised a slightly tamer circuit in the brain, ramping up our experiences of wonder, awe and elation, without tipping us into sagging sloughs of depression – would all of us queue up for it?

Were a cure for bipolar illness ever discovered, it's not clear that everyone with the diagnosis would welcome it. In surveys a majority of people with manic depression wouldn't take a cure. The Norwegian artist Edvard Munch summed up such reasoning: 'They are part of me and my art,' he wrote of his swings in mood. 'They are indistinguishable from me, and it would destroy my art. I want to keep those sufferings.'

Mania must be part of our make-up as a species – a touch of mania can help us not just individually, but as a community and society. Much has been written about how common manic-depressive illness is among creative geniuses – from Coleridge to Keats, van Gogh to Munch, Plath to Woolf – as well as among scientists. But it's unusual for someone with a severe mental illness to be able to manage to bring together the many elements required in the creation of great art – as a recent specialist review put it: 'severe psychopathology inhibits creativity. Mild and moderate disorders can inspire and motivate creative work but are only leading to new and useful solutions when creators succeed in transforming their emotional instability and cognitive incoherence into stable and coherent forms.' It's as if the tendency to mania is a scarlet thread running through the weave of our cultural heritage; without it the tapestry of our lives would be a great deal greyer, and it would be a far less imaginative world. The problem occurs when mania comes to dominate, tangling and knotting with the other threads.

We don't understand how much bipolar illness is simply inherited, how much it's an innate tendency that becomes manifest depending on exposure to stressors (upbringing, social, personal), or what the best way to treat it really is – beyond the use of drugs to even out the severity of the swings. We don't understand how a tendency to wider swings in mood than is customary (and cultures vary in their tolerance for mood swings) can sometimes be precipitated into the darker flowering of full-blown bipolar illness itself. Many of my patients with episodes of mania followed by depressed mood have learned, over years, to watch out for and avoid triggers such as overwork, sleep deprivation or stressful relationships with others; talking therapies seems to help a few identify the best ways for them to stay well. But neither drugs nor therapy are a panacea, and the potential social advantages of a scarlet thread of mania running through the weave of our communities are of little comfort when your mother or brother, uncle or niece, is running up credit card bills, driving recklessly, insulting those who care for them, drowning in self-medication.

One of my earliest lectures in psychiatry was about how to take a 'mental state examination'. As third-year medical students we had all learned how to conduct a full physical examination; now, in fourth year, we were to learn an objective approach to examining the mind. As I've emphasised throughout this book, psychiatry has none of the blood tests or scans that, in other specialties, point towards a diagnosis; even the label 'disorder' is a misnomer, given that most pathological states of mind are simply exaggerations of normal human tendencies. Instead of tests, we were taught to assess a history of the way the problem evolved, and 'examine' the mind through conversation and behaviour. The idea that diagnosis is purely on the patient's reported experience is wrong – their appearance, speech and behaviour is always part of the puzzle.

Our professor wore a brown tweed suit and matching handbag; she paced stage left to stage right, gesticulating, her dyed black hair showing ever so slightly white at the roots as she explained the importance, in writing up psychiatric notes, of creating a vivid image on paper, so that a colleague would be able to conjure the patient in their own mind's eye. The headings she told us to use were perfunctory, and followed a schema that I still use today:

Appearance (dress, hair, personal hygiene, make-up – 'and if their roots are showing,' she exclaimed, *'write that down'*);

Behaviour (agitated, subdued, body language, personal space);
Speech (content, accent, pressured, slow);
Mood (elevated, depressed, distant, engaged);
Thought (form, content, delusory, disordered);
Hallucinations (responding to unheard voices, snatching at unseen objects).

We were to gauge the patient's level of insight into their own condition, and make an estimate at their cognitive ability.

She put up a video of a man in full manic flow, showing evidence of 'tachyphrenia' (accelerated thought) and 'pressure of speech'. He was agitated and gesticulating, his eyes roved from side to side, sweat beaded on his forehead. Some of the other students laughed, perhaps from discomfort or embarrassment, because it didn't seem funny. The agitation, irritability and torment he was experiencing was palpable.

The professor went on to list some of the questions that doctors should ask in such situations, to gauge the severity of a manic episode. 'Have they been restless, unable to sleep? Have they been promiscuous or sexually disinhibited? Have they been acting impulsively? Any unwise, excessive purchases? Do they feel as if they have special powers? Have they been aggressive with friends, family or colleagues? Has there been any involvement with the police? Are there other similar episodes in their history of having been manic, high or behaving strangely? Are they experiencing any hallucinations or unusual sensations?' We were to jot all of these reflections down, and come up with a 'formulation' – elsewhere in medicine known as a 'differential diagnosis.' I was fascinated by the privilege and the licence to delve so deeply into strangers' lives that I would have to gauge how they felt and experienced the world, but at the same time unsettled that it was all so unscientific – my diagnoses were to be led by intuition and skill in communication rather than anything objective.

When someone is going high, their feeling of universal connection can spill over into elation – a state when feelings of religious illumination comes thick and fast. Here is the biologist Hope Jahren on her experience of such elation:

> You don't fear life and you don't fear death. You don't fear anything. There is no sadness and there is no grief. You feel your subconscious formulating the answers to all the collective miserable searching that man has ever done. You have indisputable proof of God and the creation of the universe. You are the one for whom the world has waited. And you will give it all back; you will pour out all you know and then wallow knee-deep in thick viscous love, love, love ... When I die I will identify Heaven only secondarily by these feelings, and primarily by their failure to end. While I am constrained to this life they will always end, and what comes after, like any resurrection, is not without cost. While this great cosmic fire hose bathes you in epiphanies, you are overtaken by your urgent need to document them and thus generate an inspired manual for all perfect tomorrows.

This blissful sense of seeing things *as they really are*, tinged with glories and beauties unavailable to the normal, everyday mind, can push sense and feeling into frank hallucination. This is the writer Jay Griffiths describing an episode of mania.

> Then I saw my wings. They were of a piece with this mad reverie: they were like a field of stars in a midnight sky. It seemed obvious that I had wings, because we all do:

wings of mind. The previous time I'd had an episode of hypomania,* I had spent a lot of time with one particular friend. I always knew he was an angel, but I had suddenly seen his wings and they were white, plump, pillowy, deep with downy feathers, as pure and healing as sleep.

For Griffiths, what had been a state of awe, elation and wonder flipped into an awe-full place where the edges of reality became blurred and the faces of friends and relatives began to show not amusement, or excitement, but concern. One of the most assiduous and careful travellers into this state of manic psychosis is Kay Redfield Jamison, a professor of psychiatry at Johns Hopkins in Baltimore and a dedicated field reporter who has brought back accounts of some of the most extreme landscapes of the mind. In her book *An Unquiet Mind* Redfield Jamison describes first the beauty and exhilaration of feeling high.

> When you're high it's tremendous. The ideas and feelings are fast and frequent like shooting stars, and you follow them until you find better and brighter ones. Shyness goes, the right words and gestures are suddenly there, the power to captivate others a felt certainty. There are interests found in uninteresting people. Sensuality is pervasive and the desire to seduce and be seduced irresistible. Feelings of ease, intensity, power, well-being, financial omnipotence and euphoria pervade one's marrow.

But then Jamison moves on to describe the darker side of mania, when it tips over into damage and destruction of

---

* 'Hypomania' is one psychiatric term for a manic episode considered to be a notch below dangerous.

relationships, of finances, risking the integrity of body and mind.

> But, somewhere, this changes. The fast ideas are far too fast, and there are far too many; overwhelming confusion replaces clarity. Memory goes. Humour and absorption on friends' faces are replaced by fear and concern. Everything previously moving with the grain is now against – you are irritable, angry, frightened, uncontrollable, and enmeshed totally in the blackest caves of the mind.

One of my patients who suffered recurrent episodes of mania told me that it took her years to learn the warning signs of when her elation, her saturation in wonder, her flight of new, world-changing, unprecedented ideas, was beginning to go sour. First to go would be her sleep – she simply didn't feel as if she needed it. She'd fill pages with scribblings: lists, mind-maps and transformative proposals to solve all the problems of the world. Then the edges of her world would start to shimmer with uncertainty, she told me, as if the foundations of reality itself were trembling. As Jamison noted, the faces of friends would begin to show concern, and for her that was the most potent warning sign. 'When you're high as a kite you have to find a way of hauling yourself back to the ground,' she said. When friends started to show concern, she told me, that was 'high time' for her to grab a tent, stove, sleeping bag and a few days of food, then take herself off to the woods.

'What is so special about the woods?' I asked her.

'The only sounds there are natural ones,' she replied: 'sounds like water, birdsong, wind.' There she could immerse herself in a different rhythm of sleep and wakefulness than the distorted one of the city, which was always pulling her out to meet people, make new connections, start new projects.

Sometimes sedatives helped, to force her mind to take some sleep. 'The healing difference is the opportunity to take time and space in a place of quiet wildness, immersed in a green world, to let my own pace and my own rhythm come back to me.' It's a response to the threat of going high that wouldn't work for everyone (and requires good camping and navigation skills), but for that particular patient, working out what she needed to stay well seemed to have pulled her back from the cliff-edge of mania several times.

In 1898 a Dr D. Inglis wrote a report for the *New York Medical Journal* on a patient with a 'Remarkable Exaggeration of the Sense of Awe'. His patient was struck dumb with wonder and awe several times a day. She was well-educated, but the parts of her brain that engaged her sense-impressions seemed caught, Inglis wrote, in a mental state like that of our distant ancestors. Hers was a gift, as it brought her many moments of beauty and wonder not accessible to others. 'The average man reasons these things out,' Inglis went on, 'and, coming of generation after generation which has reasoned them out, he is born with a mind in which the fear of the great and strange forces of Nature is relatively small.' From this point of view, loss of fear of Nature has impoverished humanity.

Awe is where elation and anxiety meet: it has been characterised as 'arrested fear', in that it is a response to the manifest majesty of phenomena much greater and more powerful than humankind. The experiences that provoke awe, transposed into a more threatening situation, might provoke terror. From the beginning of its use 'awe' carried the negative sense of fear (it is related to the word for anxiety and anguish), because of its use in the Bible to describe Old Testament experiences of a threatening, overbearing God. 'Wonder', by contrast, began as something simply strange or astonishing, but gradually took on positive associations of amazement and reverence. Religion can provoke it, but so can experiences of music and art as well as natural phenomena. Several manic patients of mine have, over the years, attested to the wondrous state of mind when they begin to go high. As a state, it's probably not exclusive to us as humans: there's a video posted online by the Jane Goodall Institute that shows chimpanzees dancing with what looks like wonder as they approach a waterfall; one chimp sits in contemplation of the flowing water as if mesmerised by its beauty.

Awe forces us to see ourselves as small, even vulnerable figures in a vast world of hidden forces; it seems to take our sense of vulnerability and make of it something to cherish. It breaks into our ideas of the individual and encourages a sense of fellowship, of shared wonder in the face of the mystery of existence. Who wouldn't want to experience more in the way of awe? I sometimes feel envious of those patients whose flights of feeling have gone so high that they are living in a sustained state of wonder: every phenomenon is connected by invisible threads of destiny and purpose that only they can see; every coincidence becomes evidence of divine or supernatural involvement; unseen powers flow through the world and can be wielded through their being.

Wonder has also been defined (in the *Oxford English Dictionary*) as 'astonishment mingled with perplexity or bewildered curiosity', and the practice of medicine is stacked with wonder-full reflections. We are made of seven billion billion billion atoms. The DNA of a single human being, stretched end to end, would leave the solar system. We can hear down to the level of individual molecules jostling within the fluid of our inner ears. How we smell remains an unfathomable mystery, though is increasingly thought to be something to do with a dynamic, perhaps quantum vibration of molecules within a vast library of specialist sensors.

Our bones are stronger than reinforced concrete, and the function of our immune system (and its interaction with the microbiome within us) remains dazzlingly mysterious, though it is fundamental to sustaining life.

Through medical school lectures and seminars, my enthusiasm for studying more about the brain and mind was fuelled by successive experiences of wonder. I thought it odd that biologists and psychologists didn't have wonder as a subject of study, and asked one of the psychology tutors why not. 'Wonder isn't directly connected to survival,' he said; 'its Darwinian role is uncertain.' Which makes wonder all the more precious: driven by satisfaction, rather than by necessity.

There seems to be a harmony in the laws of physics and the flow of forces that we have an innate ability to recognise. For the science writer Rachel Carson true spirituality is something that arises from wonder at the beauty of nature; not from adherence to the dictates of old books but from the 'humble veneration of the magnificence of life'. The world is filled with beauty and magnificence, and so are the workings of our bodies and minds; a sense of wonder can reawaken us to the unlikeliness of being. Wonder fosters humility, compassion and reverence for life – the cornerstones of all the major world religions, and fundamental qualities for the effective practice of medicine.

In a paper called 'Wonder and the clinical encounter' the philosopher H. M. Evans wrote that 'medical treatment is wonder-full in its ambition and its metaphysical presumption … I propose, to doctors and others in routine clinical life, the value of an openness to wonder and to the sense of wonder.' For a jaded, burnt-out workforce, this heightened sensitivity to unlikely wonder can be restorative. Evans realised that most clinical encounters are not like those in television dramas – they're usually undramatic, and make sustained demands on the clinician for their time, attention and empathy. An openness to wonder has the power to reinvigorate a medic's imagination, pull them back from the brink of disillusion with the demands of the work, and enhance their connections to patients as fellow human beings. The family doctor and Pulitzer Prize-winning poet William Carlos Williams wrote of this power of reinvigoration, and how he was rarely exhausted by his sessions in the clinic. 'Often after I have gone into my office harassed by personal perplexities of whatever sort, fatigued physically and mentally, after two hours of intense application to the work, I came out at the finish completely rested (and I mean rested) ready to smile and to laugh as if the day were just starting.'

The absence of wonder doesn't imply a clinical disorder the way an absence of empathy, or happiness, or caution does. Two thousand years ago, Hindu tradition placed wonder at the core of our humanity, as one of the irreducible emotions. In the early seventeenth century Thomas Browne could write, 'We carry with us the wonders we seek without us. There is all Africa and her prodigies in us.' His contemporary Descartes was the last major philosopher in the western tradition to include wonder in his list of elemental emotions. Through the 1700s something changed: the pursuit of knowledge became more structured, more effective, more international, but it also hardened, and in doing so wonder lost its central place as a human faculty, and became a kind of added extra – fuel for genius, rather than for daily life. But just as seeking out experiences of wonder might help us to flourish in life, so those experiences might help us to cherish the flourishing of the planet.

Encounters with mania have always left me wondering how it would be to be manic all of life, with no bank account or social relationships to hold you back. To fly free on glorious, exhilarating, tumultuous flurries of ideas and visionary experiences, to never come down. Would you miss peace of mind? Is a mental state even possible which combines elation with ease of being? I sometimes envy my patients the rush of it, the energising levity, but not the terror of careering out of control.

To set about healing the mind, to immerse oneself in problems of mood, is to confront the opposites we hold within us: blinding light and fathomless dark; nature seething with life and the void, empty and forever still; up and down, everything and nothing.

9

TEARS BLUE, AND WITH A WOUNDED HEART: ON DEPRESSION, MELANCHOLIA AND SUICIDE

It is wrong to believe that unmixed joy is the normal state of sensibility. Man could not live if he were entirely impervious to sadness.

Emile Durkheim

In general practice the patients tumble through the clinic like coins from a slot machine – so many! Thousands of stories glittering with the many paths to happiness or unhappiness, with the infinitude of choices, actions and reactions that make a life. To one side of my GP clinic was the richest street in the city; on the other, one of the poorest. The democratising effect of our waiting room was evident: bankers waiting side by side with heroin addicts, kids privileged by private nursery playing alongside kids who rarely got breakfast.

It was a year or two into my work there that I discovered the necessity of riding my bike the dozen miles to clinic: after a pedalling commute my mind could attend to patients and their stories with more clarity. Becoming more aware of the role of chance in how our lives turn out, for good or for bad, I found myself saying 'Good luck!' at the end of many of my consultations. Seeing patients rich and poor, it became obvious that happiness is not a simple consequence of good circumstances. Low mood and anxiety at times seemed like a barometer of the pressures being placed on the community, but it always surprised me how resilient most people are, coping with the most extraordinary difficulties. 'Shit life syndrome' is real, and ubiquitous; prosperous people have consistently better mental health than the poor as you'd expect – but wealth is no panacea. Those patients who lived in mansions, with second homes and two skiing holidays a year, complained less often of unhappiness than those on benefits – but many of them were still miserable.

Antidepressants don't figure much in the many conversations I have with people who find themselves living at the milder end of the spectrum of human unhappiness. What seems to matter is the opportunity to be listened to somewhere set apart from home, work and daily life – the separate space of the consulting room. What the GP, counsellor or therapist offer is the protected, confidential place to meet with someone who has known many others who have experienced similar states of mind, who is bound to confidentiality, and who will be able to say, 'You're not going mad.' One of its greatest gifts is the opportunity to be heard, and to be granted a fresh perspective on your troubles. Sometimes drugs are prescribed not because of the *DSM* or *ICD*, but because they may take the edge off someone's distress, and allow them the headspace to make changes that will ultimately accelerate their recovery. Much of the benefit of such drugs has been shown to be placebo. The power to sign someone off work, or write a letter to an employer or tutor, can be more transformative in easing the pressures that have contributed to reaching a crisis.

Conversations about unhappiness often circle around the social world that sustains us: fractious relationships, irritations and disappointments, work worries, relationship difficulties (whether partners or lovers, children or siblings). A GP friend of mine calls early consultations about low mood 'fishing trips': he casts his line into the lives and stories of his patients, trying to hook details of their motivations and frustrations, find out what nourishes and refreshes them, what they used to love about life but have lost. What evolves through those conversations (if they're effective) is a personal relationship. It's not entirely clear to me how often the suggestions and reflections I offer, tailored to each person's character and life experiences, are the aspect of the consultation that makes the greatest difference, or whether it's simply the opportunity to be attentively heard.

The latest iteration of the *DSM* suggests 'depression' for anyone who has suffered more than a fortnight of relentless low mood for most of the day. It asks whether someone has lost the ability to take pleasure in, or interest in, their usual activities. It asks about weight loss or weight gain, appetite loss or appetite gain, insomnia or too much sleep. When mood swings low, thoughts can slow down, and the body seems to close in on itself with a diminution in physical movement, exhaustion, fatigue. For many, that drop in vitality is accompanied by a diminution in self-worth, feeling that you're without value and, in more severe cases, unjustifiably guilty. There can be an inability to concentrate or think clearly, as well as indecisiveness. Relentless feelings of guilt and worthlessness may dovetail with recurrent thoughts of doing harm to yourself, or even killing yourself. This motley list of ghastly thoughts and feelings mean that it's quite possible for two people to be formally diagnosed with depression but have *no symptoms in common*. It's clear that 'depression' doesn't work as a discrete category, but is a catch-all term for a variety of different states of mind. It's also perfectly possible to feel happy and unhappy at the same time.

People don't come into the clinic labelled as sad, unhappy,

hopeless, despairing, despondent, suicidal; these are all words and labels that get applied through conversation and storytelling. Sometimes they're more helpful than the label 'depression', sometimes they're not. And what gets labelled 'depression' is culturally determined – studies have found that only around 3 per cent of Japanese people meet criteria for a degree of depression, compared with 17 per cent of Americans, and 18 per cent of French people. Latitude matters – if you live high in the northern hemisphere you're more likely to suffer from a seasonal depression; the formal diagnosis of seasonal affective disorder (SAD) requires that mood plummets, usually through the winter, on at least two consecutive years. It is thought to affect around 3 per cent of the UK population, though most people who experience this don't go near the doctor. Culture matters, particularly if there's discord between your own personality type and the priorities of the prevailing culture around you. An American study found that in Boston, to have a collectivist mindset which opposed individualism was associated with low mood; in Turkey, the opposite happened: people who were individualistic were more likely to be depressed. It's as if well-being is partly dependent on a synergy between your own preferred approach to life and the approach of the society around you. In India, *ashaktapana* describes a syndrome of low energy, fatigue and withdrawal; similarly in China *shenjing shuairuo* manifests bodily with weakness, fatigue, headaches, dizziness and upsets to the digestion. The 'Chinese Classification of Mental Disorders' lists types of neurasthenia, depression and anorexia which are unrecognised in the West. In Iran 'depression' is often characterised by headache, irritability and pain rather than by low mood.

'There are several languages where no words describing depression exist,' Dinesh Bhugra, a professor of Cultural Psychiatry, has noted.

However, all cultures have words describing the sadness, tiredness, lack of energy, low mood and other symptoms that constitute the constellation of depression ... When a group of Punjabi women in London were interviewed, they demonstrated quite clearly that they understood the concept of depression, including its symptoms, but they were also very clear that they would seek help from religious sources such as temples and gurudwaras because depression was part of life and not a medical problem.

Textbooks define 'depression' as more than two weeks of relentless low mood, poor self-esteem, loss of pleasure in ordinarily pleasurable things. It's a low bar, and if you questioned everyone in a typical medical waiting room, nearly one in five would meet it. As an experience it's rife: just over one in ten of the population, in any one year, could meet a diagnosis of 'major depression' according to current DSM or ICD criteria.

It can be helpful to externalise that sense of gloom: visualising it as a monkey on your back, or a charm that can be dispelled, a burden that can be thrown off. Some languages describe moods as something that descend on us, rather than as elements of our core self, and that visualisation of the mood as something that can be cast aside too can be helpful. There are other ways to imagine depressive feelings: Winston Churchill notoriously characterised his depressions as a black dog – one ordinarily kept walking to heel, but which from time to time would manage to get off its lead and cause havoc in his life. I've known people see their depressions as fogs to be blown away, as valleys of misery to be traversed. However they're imagined, seeing those episodes as changeable, outside oneself and, crucially, beatable, can be the first step to getting free of them. The reality for anyone in the grips of a major depression is that channelling positive feelings is difficult; we have to find ways of reminding ourselves that no matter how bad things get, there's always hope that they might change for the better.

'Sad, sorrowful, afflicted with low spirits' says the dictionary under *blue* – not connected to the colour's association with *movies*, with *politics* or with the *police*, but with a temporary kind of madness. It's a lengthy association, more than 500 years old – Chaucer wrote of sadness with 'tears blue, and with a wounded heart'. For a long time being *blue* explicitly meant the kind of crash in mood that happens after an alcoholic binge. *Blue devils* were those tormenting spirits that descended on an alcoholic deprived of his or her habitual poison.

It's not unusual for someone to complain of a sadness that descended, so to speak, *out of the blue*, usually accompanied by a collapse in the pleasure they're able to take in what they used to enjoy, a sense of lassitude, fogged mind, pervasive exhaustion. Overwhelmed by challenges they would once have met with ease, even with pleasure, they might take to their beds to hide from the world – though once they've retreated beneath the covers that sense of misery only deepens. And sadness is often accompanied by agitation and difficulty concentrating, the mind jittering from one distressing and depressing thought to another, without relief. There's a stamp of solemnity about the term 'depression', whereas 'the blues' implies something gentler, more fluid, transient and therefore more tolerable: as if, were we able to hold on long enough, it would flow on like water – the feeling would transform into something else.

For as long as humans have been writing we can find expressions of sadness. For much of the last couple of thousand years in the West, to be unhappy was to have an excess of black bile, or *melancholia*. Theories of sadness evolved: for much of the twentieth century, feeling blue was explained by psychoanalysts as the fallout of unconscious conflicts, childhood neglect and life dissatisfactions, all of which may be true, but didn't explain why many people who suffer equally difficult conflicts, equally neglectful childhoods and equally dissatisfying lives frequently didn't suffer from sadness much at all. The same wind blows on all of us – why are only some of us flattened by it?

The earliest antidepressant pills were tuberculosis (TB) antibiotics. Before modern therapies became available through the 1950s and 1960s, sufferers of TB would be sequestered for months, even years, in institutions built at altitude, with seated terraces exposed to frigid winds (the breathing of cold air deep into the lungs was thought to slow, even reverse, infection). People committed to an institution often became depressed at being cooped up for months, trapped by disease. When the first antituberculosis drugs were invented, reports began to emerge of withdrawn melancholic patients dancing between their beds. Perhaps those drugs really did have an effect on the mind, but hope too can be a powerful drug. We no longer use antituberculosis drugs to treat mood (their success was overstated), and by the mid-1960s they were superseded by another class of drugs derived from antihistamines. Pharmaceutical companies like to characterise antidepressants as in some way specific to mood, but that's not true. Most were invented for something else, and their effect on mood is a side effect that we have slowly learned how to harness.

The first widely available psychiatric drug derived from antihistamines was a major tranquilliser, chlorpromazine, which was so commercially successful that pharmaceutical companies began to experiment with minor modifications to its structure. After a great deal of trial and error, and the endurance of harrowing side effects on the part of study participants, one of these tweaked drugs, called imipramine, was found to have an elevating effect on mood. At the time of its invention in the mid-twentieth century many psychiatrists still characterised sadness in Freudian terms, as the result of unconscious conflicts and frustrations. Antidepressant drugs were not then prescribed to treat the *cause* of low mood, only to help mitigate its effects while the patient embarked on psychotherapy. Offering the drugs was, for these Freudian-minded psychiatrists, like giving paracetamol for fever, or antihistamines for itch – a symptomatic treatment while the real work of healing went on elsewhere.

These drugs never needed to have a *specific* antidepressant effect to be thought of as helpful. If your preponderant emotion is one of bleak futility and despair, any drug that can blunt intensity of emotional feeling is to be welcomed. But then once the blackness has retreated, the same drug might be unwelcome because it also distances you from pleasurable, rewarding emotions.

Marketing for these new drugs played its part in their great success through the 1960s. In 1961, when Ken Kesey was writing *One Flew Over the Cuckoo's Nest*, amitriptyline was approved for use and began to be marketed as a safe alternative to electro-convulsive therapy (ECT). Its manufacturer Merck commissioned a Baltimore psychiatrist to write a short giveaway manual for physicians called *Recognizing the Depressed Patient: with essentials of management and treatment*. It was the era of Arthur C. Clarke, Robert Heinlein and Isaac Asimov; of Yuri Gagarin orbiting the planet in Vostok 1. It was believed that technology would deliver us into a glorious new future free of human unhappiness; pills would banish the age-old miseries of mankind. Fifty thousand of Merck's manuals were distributed for free, and another hundred thousand copies were sold to a public eager to understand this exciting new dawn: psychopharmacology.

Within twenty years it was possible to be sued as a doctor for *not* prescribing antidepressants.

By the 1990s Prozac and its siblings were lucrative beyond the most outrageous projections of the companies' marketing departments. But as orders for more and more similar drugs soared, the results began to come in: for low mood at the milder end of the spectrum (what we might still call *the blues*) these newer antidepressant drugs *didn't work at all*. Around 90 per cent of any positive effect they might have was down to the placebo effect.

Placebos are the most studied drug in history – every new medication is trialled against them. Their power is well-documented: the new antidepressant pills looked modern, sophisticated, specific. They had been greatly hyped, and both doctor and patient believed in them. But significant in their success was that they also made you feel slightly strange; this 'enhanced placebo' effect gave them a better chance of working than inert pills. Recipients complained of loose bowels, sleepless nights, a collapse in libido. That the drugs clearly had the power to influence such primitive aspects of our humanity as sleep, digestion and sex meant it became easier to believe they had substantial power over the mind too. One advantage Prozac held over the older antidepressants was that people taking it seemed more likely to lose weight than to gain it; another advantage was that if someone happened to overdose on it, they were more likely to survive.

Antidepressants save lives, but for the majority of people suffering from low mood they do little good at all – in fact they're potentially harmful, because they dupe the taker into thinking they have some biochemical imbalance that can only be corrected through dependency on medication. There are some studies that suggest that taking antidepressants actually slows recovery. Eighty-five per cent of depressions that are untreated recover on their own within twelve months, while recovery rates from *treated* depressions can be as low as 22 per cent. A 2023 study published in the prestigious journal *Molecular Psychiatry* reviewed all the evidence, and concluded: 'the huge research effort based on the serotonin hypothesis has not produced convincing evidence of a biochemical basis to depression ... We suggest it is time to acknowledge that the serotonin theory of depression is not empirically substantiated.'

There are billions of reasons for feeling low – as many reasons as there are people. And there are millions of people who feel low from time to time for no identifiable reason at all. Sadness can be caused by not getting enough light in the winter, by grief, by creeping life dissatisfactions, disappointments, abuse, by loss of status, dysfunctional relationships, frustrated ambitions. It can be caused by shitty jobs, overpowering addictions, overbearing neighbours or colleagues and substandard housing. And the answers to those problems, in all of those situations, must necessarily include addressing those triggers themselves.

How to light a candle to dispel the gloom? There are some for whom it's enough to be really heard – listened to, not judged – by family, friends or some kind of counselling or medical professional. Feeling oneself part of humanity, rather than isolated and alone, is about as therapeutic a sensation as it's possible to have, and many of my patients have found relief from depression through building networks of friends into therapeutic communities, whether explicitly or subconsciously.

It doesn't seem to matter whether someone engages in family systems theory or Gestalt, psychoanalysis or CBT, or whether they access counselling through a specialist counsellor or a psychiatrist, a mental health nurse or a GP. One study from the 1960s compared the results of senior experienced psychotherapists with laypeople (the language of the day called them 'housewives') who had undergone just a couple of years' training: it found that the laypeople's results were as good as the psychotherapists. If someone is unwell they'd be well advised to find someone they trust, to talk about their feelings, and that trust is the basis of recovery. It's not always necessary to reach for the drugs and a therapist: get the basics right first – a set of lanterns that will help guide the way through the darker places of the mind.

All of us need sleep, and good-quality sleep. Switching off screens in the evening, avoiding caffeine after 4 p.m., getting a comfortable bed, avoiding working or snacking in bed, keeping it dark, no naps through the day, winding down gently in the evenings – all these help make sure that when the time comes to sleep, your chance of drifting off is at its best.

Move: the body knows how to live, and so using that body every day to get some exercise, to the best of someone's ability or disability, helps. Even in significant depressions the effect of half an hour of exercise a day, vigorous enough to get out of breath, is proven to be as good for your mood as a prescription of antidepressants. Exercise makes the mind feel better through hormonal changes of the body, as well as allowing it time to switch off.

Finding a community helps – even the most cantanker-ous misanthrope among us is, at root, a social human being. Working on connections with old friends helps too, as does joining groups and clubs of people that share enthusiasms (and seeking out new ones). Human beings are social beings, and benefit from finding ways to share and connect with others. Volunteering improves levels of happiness, and seems to have an effect on general physical health too. Having a reason to get out and be with others can seem an impossi-ble obstacle for some, but can offer a sense of purpose and value to life. If disappointments, conflicts and relationships are the problem, counselling can help: there's no substitute for being heard and having an experienced listener help you gather perspective and fresh ideas.

If depressive feelings are brought on by the miserable, cold darkness of a northern winter, it's worth getting as much light through the day as possible, even if it's artificial light (though light from the sky is best). Spending time with loved ones can be a tonic, bringing back into focus those aspects of life most worth cherishing – relationships. It's not possible to will yourself into faith, but it's notable that people who regularly attend religious services have over 20 per cent lower rates of depression and low mood than those who don't, at least in part because of the supportive benefits of a shared community.

Almost everyone can think of something that gives them pleasure, that used to make them feel good before they began to feel so bad, something that nourishes their sense of well-being and makes them feel more alive. When the philosopher David Hume felt low, he wrote that he'd get away from his books, take himself out for a fine meal with friends, play backgammon, laugh and joke with others in company. More on him in a moment, but his suggestion to do more of the things that make you feel good, and less of the things that make you feel tense, stressed, sad and disappointed, remains wise advice. We don't have control over many of the events of our lives, but we do have control over how we respond to them.

For some people antidepressant drugs will play a role, though after decades and billions of dollars-worth of research, their role remains uncertain. They all have side effects: nausea, loose bowels, dry mouth, insomnia, collapsing libido, but for many of my patients those side effects are a small price to pay for the chance of feeling better. There are three main classes of antidepressants, and a good rule is that if something was helpful in the past, it's worth trying again. I'm often asked by patients how quickly, after they start feeling well, they can reduce their dose: though everyone is different, it's a good idea to have at least three months of feeling relatively well before discussing a reduction with whoever is prescribing it. Even then it's something I'd suggest only tentatively, and be ready to increase the dose again if necessary.

There's a view that life's ups and downs will eventually balance out – and for some people that seems to be true: if for a while their mood has been going down, they wait it out, and they'll soon be due an up. Even the most severe depressive illnesses have a natural course and, given enough time, they often pass – if stressors and provoking factors can ease. Following advice, speaking with someone trustworthy, considering medication and holding fast will see many people all right in the end. The gloom may come back, but next time they'll be better prepared.

Once upon a time there was a worry that to ask someone about his or her suicidal feelings would trigger the act – as if suicide wasn't already dominant in the mind of someone pushed to such an extreme. But the reverse is true: talking about feelings of despair can help, and won't make someone more likely to seek out their own death. But to ask someone if they're contemplating suicide is a hard conversation to start. Responses vary: for some it's a relief to articulate their misery, for others it remains unvoiced because it's unvoiceable.

To doubt there's meaning or worth in life is to challenge the sense of meaning or worth in anyone's life. A therapist faced with a suicidal patient is asked to confront the question, however subliminally: what is the value of life? To comfort someone in such despair it becomes necessary to voice the conviction that life has meaning, even if that meaning has been temporarily obscured, or fogged, or thrown off track, by a shift in that person's state of mind. A way out is to offer reassurance that enjoyment in life can return, does return, that the therapist has seen it return again and again. To offer hope.

In his memoir of depression *Darkness Visible* the writer William Styron described in forensic detail the feeling of melancholia sliding towards suicide. There are many such accounts, but Styron's is particularly elegant in capturing the devastation of severe depression, and how inadequate the word 'depression' is as a descriptor of such a state of mind.

> 'Melancholia' would still appear to be a far more apt and evocative word for the blacker forms of the disorder, but it was usurped by a noun with a bland tonality and lacking any magisterial presence, used indifferently to describe an economic decline or a rut in the ground, a true wimp of a word for such a major illness ... for over seventy-five years the word has slithered innocuously through the language like a slug, leaving little trace of its intrinsic malevolence and preventing, by its very insipidity, a general awareness of the horrible intensity of the disease when out of control.

Styron lost his mother as a boy, and his book describes a series of midlife triggers for what became, for him, the disintegration of his sense of self. When he reached the point where his own bath seemed nothing more than a receptacle for opening his veins, the rafters in his loft simply scaffolds for a rope, he went to his lawyer to finalise a will and prepare for suicide:

> the gray drizzle of horror induced by depression takes on the quality of physical pain. But it is not an immediately

identifiable pain, like that of a broken limb. It may be more accurate to say that despair, owing to some evil trick played upon the sick brain by the inhabiting psyche, comes to resemble the diabolical discomfort of being imprisoned in a fiercely overheated room. And because no breeze stirs this cauldron, because there is no escape from this smothering confinement, it is entirely natural that the victim begins to think ceaselessly of oblivion.

What he needed was not oblivion, or even a cure for melancholia, but to get himself to a place of safety. 'I could not commit this desecration on myself,' he wrote, and immediately sought help. Antidepressants are only partially useful, he added, comparing them to the flimsy attempts to treat infection that prevailed before antibiotics were invented.

The hospital to which Styron was admitted for seven weeks was a grim place of locked doors and soulless corridors, but its very separation from the world of comfort and routine was, he wrote, his salvation. The knives of his own kitchen – glittering and seductive – had been replaced by flimsy ones of institutional plastic. The routines of the hospital, its 'orderly and benign detention', were experienced as a framework in which his mind could rest and find its own ways to heal. A sedative hitherto prescribed by his psychiatrist was stopped and the urgency of his suicidal feelings began to recede. He wondered if the drug itself had been worsening his warped frame of mind. His body, which had felt like a desiccated husk, began to feel vivid again, as if the juices within it were stirring. For months sleep had been dreamless, but strange, symbolic dreams of birds and dancers began to return. Light began to penetrate the darkness of his mind: 'For me the real healers were seclusion and time.'

Too often we've lost this sense of the psychiatric hospital as *asylum*, as a place of safety. When only the most extreme, chaotic and violent patients are admitted, the majority are left to seek their own forms of sanctuary elsewhere.

Hamlet's 'To be or not to be' was largely rhetorical in Shakespeare's day – suicide was forbidden by God and suicide was worse than murder. The impulse for self-annihilation was to be deterred rather than treated with compassion: the bodies of suicides were tossed on the town midden, buried at crossroads with stakes through their hearts, and in France, under Louis XVI, dragged across town face down through the dust. That suicide implied abject moral degradation was taken for granted when David Hume proposed the contrary view in his essay *On Suicide* – which was published only after his death in 1776. Hume argued of suicide that 'we may at least be assured that any one who, without apparent reason, has had recourse to it, was cursed with such an incurable depravity or gloominess of temper as must poison all enjoyment, and render him equally miserable as if he had been loaded with the most grievous misfortunes.'

There's a lot hanging on Hume's use of 'incurable'. When I frame suicidal feelings as a passing storm, an illness to be treated, an irrational conviction to be reasoned away, it's buttressed with the memory of many recoveries I've seen over decades of practice. Supportive community, and prompt access to psychiatric services, can both help. Hume's essay assumed that 'gloominess of temper' was something unamenable to treatment, but we know the reverse is true.

For a while now I've been asking therapists about suicides among their patients. It helps me in thinking about my own, as I pick endlessly over the antecedents of each, wondering whether there was something I missed. There's often a solemn and melancholic air to that conversation with fellow therapists, a kind of wistful regret mixed with puzzlement, as slowly each begins to talk, to remember, to ask themselves whether anything else might have been done. I've asked GPs, counsellors, psychoanalysts and psychiatrists, impressed but not surprised by the detail with which each story is recounted, even decades after the event. They remember the cast of light at their last conversation with the deceased, their particular facial expression, the tone of voice on the last answerphone message. The suicides I've known have been broadly representative of the phenomenon: mostly men, who've mostly chosen violent deaths, mostly coming from deprived or oppressed communities. About three-quarters of suicides are male. Half of all suicides in the world take place in China and in India, though those countries make up only about a quarter of the world's population.

I'm haunted by the memory of my last meeting with a broken-hearted young call-centre worker, barely able to speak because talking would involve a pause in the frantic checking of his phone for messages that didn't come. I made soothing reassurances, offered a prescription to dull his agitation, a referral, and arranged a review later in the week that he didn't attend. I followed up by phone, but couldn't reach him – three weeks later he took his own life. The woman disabled by multiple sclerosis who took an overdose, then put a bag over her head. The soldier who hiked out onto the moor, lay down in the heather, and overdosed. The sociologist Emile Durkheim theorised as to why suicide is so common among military personnel – not simply because of the devastating effects of war, or because of their easy access to weapons, but because of the depersonalising effect of army training: 'Military esprit can only be strong if the individual is self-detached, and such detachment necessarily throws the door open to suicide.'

I remember too, with more gladness, the man who climbed a tree in his garden with the intention of hanging himself, and jumped. The branch broke, and he fell to the earth as if reborn – those lungfuls of grassy air tasted sweet, he said, and he has never contemplated his own death again. Most had never spoken to me of their plans – the Samaritans estimate only half of UK suicides have ever had any contact with mental health services, and the police report on the desk can be my first intimation of such despair. These episodes are remembered so vividly in part because suicides are rare – I can count those I've known in thirty years of practice on just a couple of hands. But suicide's seismic aftermath reverberates on through the years; although the acts themselves might be sporadic, the misery they cause may become routine clinical fare, going on through the decades, spreading through families, undermining relationships, setting off aftershocks. A therapist might know only a few clients or patients who have died by suicide, but will have had scores of patients struggling with the grief of having lost a friend or relative to suicide.

And those relatives and friends are often the strongest protective factors against it. I've known dozens of people who have told me that the only thing that's keeping them from attempting suicide themselves is the knowledge of what such a violent departure would do to their loved ones. And pets, of course; I remember one woman for whom the decision to live or die came down to the simple question: who would look after the cats?

To feel depressed about the state of your life is to demonstrate the capacity to imagine something different, and that spark of imagination can prove a motive to change. Often in the clinic I find myself reminding my own patients that they're not alone in feeling down or despairing; it just feels that way – a large proportion of those who claim volubly to be enjoying life are faking it. Social media has extended this kind of deception, but behind the closed clinic door you see a different picture of humanity, one broken but with the capacity to mend, one that struggles on against unspoken difficulties, often with great courage.

When I think of the hundreds of patients I've heard speak of suicide over the last three decades, whether their own or that of others, and I imagine all those I'll no doubt hear in the years of medical practice to come, what seems most of help is not an unwarranted optimism, or a belief that suicide can be right or that it is always wrong, but our flawed human capacity to hold mutually contradictory beliefs and voice them with conviction. When the task in hand is to convince a suicidal patient there's value and purpose in life, then thoughts of suicide are best framed as a shared enemy, a corruption of reality, a manifestation of illness – something to be reasoned away, or quelled with medication. But for the families of the dead, who sit later in the same consulting room, those metaphors of distortion and disease can be unhelpful, even hurtful, and what best replaces them are metaphors of victory and redemption, of suffering followed by release.

Psychological studies of Buddhist monks have shown that those who meditate have access to a mood that is neither high nor low, but is felt as a blissful, balanced equanimity. 'Meditation mitigated depressive mood, anger, hostility and fatigue and increased vigour,' reported one study, conducted with monks in Japan and Myanmar. '[M]editation enables people to control their emotions and feelings, and, as the years of experience of meditation increase, meditation may enhance the ability (psychological flexibility) to find what is important for their present self without worrying about incidents of the past and uncertainty of the future.'

There's a famous Buddhist parable in which a warrior on a battlefield, struck by an arrow, begins to ask, 'Who shot this arrow? Where was it made? Of what is it composed?' instead of simply pulling the arrow out. Caught in a rising tide of despair, many people get stuck with questions such as, 'How deep will this go?' 'Why now?' 'How did I get here?', when the urgent matter is to get back onto dry land.

Many voice their experience of lowering despair in stark, life-or-death terms – 'sinking in a mire', 'hammered by life', 'trapped in a fire'. The place of safety or escape from that torment might be different for everyone, but it's of paramount necessity to find it. Just as William Styron saw hospital as an asylum, or place of safety, so it's important to remove the demands of home and of work (unless work itself is restorative and refreshing). Eating well, and doing all that's possible to promote restful sleep, is worthwhile, as is disconnection from online 'compare-and-despair' social media worlds of shaming and indignation. Styron noted too that it was necessary to forget about urgency of recovery – these things take their own time. A notice in my consulting room offers a ten-point plan for a flourishing mind and mood.

1. Learn something
2. Think of good things you've done
3. Take care of what you eat
4. Keep in touch with friends and loved ones
5. Keep physically active
6. Be kind to yourself
7. Get involved and make a contribution
8. Take a break
9. Ask for help and share what you're feeling
10. Make something!

It's difficult to live in a place of cold, empty sadness, but the statistics suggest that for most of us, it will pass.

10

PRIVY TO A DREAM: ON PSYCHOSIS, DELUSIONS AND HALLUCINATIONS

The enduring and pervasive feeling of being unreal
is the disease itself. When I realised this condition
was permanent, to perceive myself as in a movie, I
understood it would eventually destroy the core of
my life.

Patient quoted by Ragnhild Husby and Paul Møller in
The Initial Prodrome in Schizophrenia

Low. High. Anxious. Traumatised. These are feelings anybody can relate to. When they arrive at the doors of a clinic
it is because of the distress they cause. And the boundaries
between them are often blurred: anxiety and low mood often
march together because of the way they feed on one another
in a mind that overthinks. Within limits, high and low mood
are part of the cycles of life, and I've yet to meet someone
whose mood is relentlessly level. Anyone who has ever been
neglected, humiliated, victimised and traumatised may suffer from aspects of thinking, feeling and being that go to the
core of who they are, and whether they can feel safe,
grounded in the world and in relationships. As a general
practitioner I encounter these problems every day, and in the
old days they would all be characterised as 'neurotic'. People

suffering a neurosis are inhabiting the same perceptual world as everyone else, but certain aspects of feeling have been heightened to a pitch of anguish.

'Psychosis' is another state of mind entirely, in which the bonds of reality seem to have slipped. Sufferers have beliefs that are manifestly untrue (delusions), or perceptions that are manifestly not there (hallucinations). *Delusion* comes from the Latin word for deception, or being deceived; *hallucination* comes from the Latin *alucinatus*, meaning to wander in the mind or to dream.

At any waking moment there are thousands of possible sensations, memories and visualisations to which it's possible for the mind to attend; reality isn't presented to us through our senses as established fact; we weave it in part from our perceptions, and in part from our expectations and memories. In psychosis the balance has shifted so far towards expectation (or fear) that the fabric of reality itself starts to unravel. Someone with a manic psychosis may really *see* wings on their angelic friend; someone with psychotic depression may really believe that they have died and are rotting inside. When recurrent psychosis is equally mingled with disturbance of mood, it is called 'schizoaffective disorder'.

In Esmé Weijun Wang's memoir of schizoaffective disorder, *The Collected Schizophrenias*, she writes, 'Should delusion come to call, or hallucinations crowd my senses again, I might be able to wrangle sense out of the senseless. I tell myself that if I must live with a slippery mind, I want to know how to tether it too.' Her book is in part an enquiry into the question of what can hold the mind together when reality itself starts to fall to pieces.

Hearing voices is a common hallucination in psychosis; 75 per cent of people diagnosed as schizophrenic hear voices of one kind or another. But voice-hearing itself is not necessarily pathological – up to one in ten people hear voices from time to time, and for some people, inner dialogues and reflections can start to be perceived as voices. A ten-year research project at Durham University ('Hearing the Voice') concluded, 'Voice-hearing experiences are fairly common and not necessarily a cause for concern. If you find that these experiences continue to cause significant distress or interfere with your relationships or daily activities, you should seek the advice of your GP.' Socrates reportedly heard voices, as did Martin Luther King and Sigmund Freud. It's when those voices cause distress or disturbance that those experiences cross the line into clinical disorder.

For decades, orthodox psychiatry has for good reason focused on quietening the psychotic mind with sedatives, a class of drugs still known as 'major tranquillisers'. But in recent years a radical new treatment for psychotic hallucinations has been developed, in which the human capacity to hear voices is turned to the sufferers' advantage. Researchers at King's College London have been testing a new 'AVATAR therapy', where voice hearers have the opportunity to build and then converse with an animated digital representation of the distressing voice they hear. In truth it's another kind of talking therapy, but instead of talking directly to the patient, the trained therapist talks through the 'avatar', mimicking the hateful or distressing voice with software so that the patient can learn techniques of naming and then standing up to domineering voices. It is still early days in this treatment, but some researchers at King's College London are optimistic: 'Over the course of [brief or extended] versions of the therapy, the avatar comes to recognise the voice hearer's strengths and good qualities, becomes less hostile, and concedes power to them,' they explained. It can be transformative, putting agency and autonomy back into a situation characterised by weakness and vulnerability. 'I remember walking home from that session with a smile on

my face. Something had shifted,' wrote one of the participants; 'my confidence began to grow. I was also able to start
putting some boundaries in place with my voices in my daily
life.'

The propensity for madness is an ancient aspect of our
humanity, commented on in the earliest literature we know
of: from the Bible's Nebuchadnezzar, who eats grass and
believes himself to be a beast, to Herodotus's Cleomenes,
who in a fit of madness sliced muscles from his own legs.
One of the earliest modern accounts of psychosis is John
Haslam's *Illustrations of Madness: exhibiting a singular case of
insanity, and a no less remarkable difference in medical opinion
developing the nature of assailment and the manner of working
events*. It was published in 1810; the patient was James Tilly
Matthews, who had been admitted to London's Bethlem
('Bedlam') asylum in January 1797. He believed that a 'gang
of villains, profoundly skilled in pneumatic chemistry', was
attacking him; 'while one of these villains is sucking out the
brain of the person assailed, to extract his existing sentiments, another of the gang will force into his mind a train of
ideas very different from the real subject of his thoughts.'
Matthews also described 'sudden death squeezing, stomach
skinning, apoplexy making with the nutmeg grater, length-
ening of the brain, thought making and laugh making'.

Matthews clearly had a set of delusional beliefs and perceptions, and a disorder of thinking. He believed his assailants
worked at a distance through something called an 'air loom'
to influence him, and this loom also communicated the voices
that he heard. (Just as today psychotic patients often believe
microchips and wi-fi are having a malign effect, so psychotic
people of the nineteenth century too imagined the sophisticated technology of their day could turn against them.) This
brief description of Matthews' delusions demonstrates most

of what the German psychiatrist Kurt Schneider much later called the 'first-rank symptoms' of schizophrenia:

- audible thoughts
- voices heard arguing
- voices heard commenting on one's actions
- the experience of influences playing on the body
- thought withdrawal and other interferences with thought
- thoughts being broadcast outside the head to others
- delusional perceptions
- feelings, impulses and volitional acts experienced as the work or influence of others

Matthews' family petitioned to have him released, and a variety of medical opinions were sought. Several physicians were found who pronounced him sane. The purpose of Haslam's account was to demonstrate that Matthews was *insane*, and that his delusions and hallucinations had not diminished during his long years held in Bedlam. 'Madness being opposite to reason and good sense as light is to darkness, straight to crooked, etc., it appears wonderful that two opposite opinions could be entertained on the subject,' Haslam wrote. Deciding which beliefs 'count' as madness and which do not is as controversial in our day as it was in 1810. Haslam's case posed the question of who can be detained against their will, for the safety of themselves and others – and it's a question that still goes to the heart of modern psychiatry.

Before the UK's Royal College of Psychiatrists took its current name it was the Royal Medico-Psychological Association. Before that it was the Association of Medical Officers of Asylums and Hospitals for the Insane. Way back in its origins, psychiatry had its roots in safety, not in the relief of distress.

Insane people were locked away for others' safety and occasionally their own. This preoccupation with safety and the
legal framework around when someone can be deprived of
their freedom because of their mental state persists into
modern medical practice. As a doctor, one of the very few
interactions I have with the law concerns the detention of
people against their will for the purposes of assessment and
treatment of mental disorder. The modern Scottish legisla-
tion goes like this:

As the medical practitioner named on page 1, I declare
that I have examined the patient. I am granting this emergency detention certificate because I believe the patient
meets the following criteria – I consider it is likely, for
the reasons stated below, that the patient has a mental
disorder ...
I consider it likely, for the reasons stated below, that
because of this mental disorder, the patient's ability to
make decisions about the provision of medical treatment for mental disorder is significantly impaired ...
I am satisfied, for the reasons stated below, that it is
necessary as a matter of urgency to detain the patient in
hospital for the purpose of determining what medical
treatment for mental disorder the patient requires ...
I am satisfied, for the reasons stated below, that if the
patient were not detained in hospital there would be a
significant risk – to the patient's health, safety or welfare
or to the safety of any other person ...
I am satisfied, for the reasons stated below, that
making arrangements with a view to the granting of a
short-term detention certificate would involve undesir-
able delay. [Give details of efforts which were made with
respect to granting a short-term detention certificate ...
Please give details of the alternatives which you

considered to the granting of this certificate. Why is informal/voluntary care not appropriate?]

Mental Health (Care and Treatment) (Scotland) Act 2003

I've signed a fair few of these emergency detention forms over the years. It's always a fraught and protracted process, with little humanity in it, and little need for the kind of labels that dominate psychiatry textbooks. To be detained it's enough to be putting yourself and others at risk, and there to be the suspicion that *you're not in your right mind,* and to be in need of further assessment by a psychiatrist.

I remember Barbara, an elderly lady who lived quietly for many years with the conviction that her neighbours stole into her house by night to move things around. The police were accustomed to her complaints. Despite numerous encounters and conversations there was nothing I could do to shift Barbara's conviction, or to help her adjust to a more reassuring reality. Her delusion was fixed, and though she was distressed by her belief, her behaviour was, ultimately, benign: she wasn't a risk to herself or others, she wasn't detainable, she wouldn't agree to meet with a psychiatrist, and I couldn't oblige her to take any medication. She had never done anything to make her neighbours afraid for their own safety, and seemed unlikely to pose a threat to them.

Another patient of mine, Richard was not so fortunate. He had been picked up many times by the police muttering about the heat, noise, concrete and metal of the cities, and knocking the wing mirrors off cars. This had frequently been an early sign of a psychotic episode, and if he wasn't admitted to psychiatric care, he would have been in police custody charged with vandalism. At such times he insisted not only that the corporate world was poison, but also that mobile phone masts were inserting thoughts into his brain and removing them from it. Aged twenty-seven, he had been homeless for a while. I asked him, when he was relatively well, how he spent his days, and he told me that he walked more than twenty miles a day, sleeping wherever he found himself when tired. When he started to become more unwell the women he passed on the street all had his mother's face. If the hospital ward phone rang an even number of times it would be his real father who had made the call, but if it rang an odd number of times, a doppelgänger.

He filled pages with dense scribbles that were illegible to me, but which I longed to decipher. He often appeared to be listening and responding to voices that I couldn't hear. One day he escaped the ward and walked miles out to the periphery of the city, only to orbit back again by evening, to willingly take his antipsychotic drugs.

He resented being held against his will. His illness struck me as a disturbing revelation of the interconnectedness of everything, patterned in complex and inscrutable ways, gone badly awry. When you realise that all things influence one another at least in small ways – butterfly wings to hurricanes, experiences to feelings – it's just a small step towards the conviction that the number of times a phone rings determines who it will be on the other end of the line.

Kerry had taken a lot of drugs in the last year: LSD, cocaine, cannabis, speed. She'd been left in a terrified state: she saw trails behind fast-moving objects, the teeth of strangers appeared to chatter at her like skulls, and she felt afraid all the time.

Sometimes as sleep approached, visions came: always horrifying, oppressive and terrorising. They had some of the flavour of an acute religious experience – awe, trembling – but she also had the sense she was being infiltrated by alien minds. She would lie panting, attempting to rationalise her way out of it, her heartbeat like hooves galloping. She told me that often she'd roll over to stare at the floor until the feeling passed.

'How can you tell people,' she asked me, 'without sounding pretentious, that you have actually been to hell and back? That you've touched madness and felt what it is to lose touch with your own self? How do you tell them that your consciousness isn't reliable or stable? Our minds are nothing more than rickety scaffolding – they can fall apart any minute.'

Her grip on reality still felt shaky, and her illness heavily soaked in anxiety. At her worst times, she said, she felt like a bubble whirling in a torrential flow of thoughts. 'Sometimes even viewing a single word, a letter of the alphabet, is terrifying,' she went on. 'My mind tries to get a grip on it being two things at once – ink on paper, and a symbol with meaning – and I can't fit both those realities into my mind at once. When it's bad, even to glimpse the words on a corridor sign has me covering up my eyes.'

She was afraid of the dark, because in darkness her mind threatened to fall away into nothing. In a light space, visible objects could give her mind something to grasp onto. 'Alcohol and TV are a refuge,' she said. 'They're mindless, and are such a relief to me when my mind is working overtime, and those attacks of unreality come without any warning.' It wasn't a feeling that *nothing* was real, she explained, but instead as though nothing could ever be fixed, reliable, absolutely true, or have any firm substance.

I was reminded of the idea of the 'ground of being', and the necessity that the mind has structure, and that the structure rests on firm foundations. 'What is the mind?' she asked me. 'In those moments it's terrifying to realise that nothing is really holding it together.' If nothing anchors the ship of the mind, then, slipped from moorings, it might be free to drift away somewhere irretrievable, capsize or even sink.

Her psychiatrist didn't have many options, he said, and intended to treat Kerry with escalating doses of antipsychotics. For him every feeling and perception Kerry had told a story of aberration and deviation – there was nothing of value in her new perspective, no insights. But I had the feeling that Kerry was on a journey, and that if she could be guided gently through the frightening landscapes of her mind, perhaps by another patient who had returned from a similar state, she might return stronger, and wiser, from the experience.

In his book *The Politics of Experience* the psychiatrist Ronald Laing included this quote by Gregory Bateson about psychosis as a journey, or even pilgrimage, that so often goes wrong.

> It would appear that once precipitated into psychosis the patient has a course to run. He is, as it were, embarked upon a voyage of discovery which is only completed by his return to the normal world, to which he comes back with insights different from those of the inhabitants who never embarked on such a voyage … What needs to be explained is the failure of many who embark upon this voyage to return from it. Do these encounter circumstances either in family life or in institutional care so grossly maladaptive that even the richest and best organized hallucinatory experience cannot save them?

In the UK 13 per cent of people who have a psychotic experience that comes to the attention of psychiatry have only one episode, and no subsequent enduring illness, while 30 per cent may have several episodes, but no enduring illness. But almost 50 per cent have recurrent episodes that profoundly impact on their ability to hold down work and stable relationships, with the episodes worsening a little each time.

Part of me wondered whether getting a label of psychosis

would be helpful to Kerry. She had been tipped into madness by hallucinogenic drugs; those drugs may have uncovered an innate tendency she carried within her, but if she stayed drug-free might she not also have the chance to come back to trusting her perceptions again? Her storytelling self might have the opportunity to make sense of her experience through understanding it as an extended bad trip, rather than an irrevocable twisting of her mind. There's a view that drug-induced psychosis can 'kindle' a more enduring split from reality, as if once the mind has been so inflamed, it catches alight more readily with minimal triggers in the future. But flames can be put out: I wanted Kerry to be able to meet people who had been through similar experiences, and found ways through. From where I stood it appeared as if she was suffering from an excruciating, staggering unsteadiness of mind *revealed* by the drugs, rather than a mind which had been broken by them. A negligible distinction, perhaps, but given that part of recovery is the ability to create a story of our experience that makes sense to us, an important one.

After my conversation with Kerry I walked back with her to the main ward, the common room thick with cigarette smoke. Most of the patients were hunched in their private hells, each sucking on a cigarette as if tobacco smoke could be a substitute for mother's milk.

Alois Alzheimer was of the gilded, late nineteenth-century generation of German neuropsychiatrists; so too was Emil Kraepelin, Alzheimer's colleague, who saw mental distress as a collection of related symptoms not dissimilar from the 'network theory' of mental disorders promulgated today, in which symptoms are thought to mutually reinforce one another: e.g. social anxiety causes and reinforces withdrawn behaviour; agitation causes and reinforces insomnia.

Kraepelin was a man of his age, a racist and eugenicist,

but he also saw his patients' problems as part of a lifelong story, inflected and influenced by their backgrounds, families and individual resilience. He was anxious that psychiatry achieve parity of esteem with other medical specialties, and in his inaugural lecture as a professor, given in 1886 when he was just thirty years old, he said, 'Over the course of the last decade, psychology has become a natural science like any other, and therefore it has a legitimate right to expect that its achievements receive the same respect and recognition as other auxiliary disciplines that we use to construct our scientific house.' It's a parity that is still lacking.

He paid close attention to what his patients were experiencing, rather than simply dismissing them. He wrote that they 'see mice, ants, the hound of hell, scythes, and axes. They hear cocks crowing, shooting, birds chirping, spirits knocking, bees humming, murmurings, screaming, scolding, voices from the cellar'. He tried to make an inventory of his patients' outpourings: 'the voices say filthy things, all conceivable confused stuff, just fancy pictures; they speak about what the patient does ... They say: "That man must be beheaded, hanged," "Swine, wicked wretch, you will be done for."' He was at pains to distinguish degenerative psychosis, which so often presented with a relentless downward trajectory, from that of manic depression, or what he called 'circular insanity', with its cycling peaks and troughs of mood. He noted that the former, which he called *dementia praecox*, had worse outcomes, with little hope of restoration, as if its victims had been struck by a malign enchantment, or by lightning. *Dementia praecox* or 'precocious dementia' is a poor title for such a complex set of problems, and, sure enough, within a few years a Swiss colleague, Eugen Bleuler, came up with another title, which proved to have better stickability: schizophrenia.

As a youth Bleuler had seen his sister admitted to a

madhouse in a catatonic trance, and been horrified by the dismissive and undignified way she had been treated. He resolved to become a psychiatrist and prove that a better way was possible. He coined his famous term from the Greek *schizo*, for 'split', and *phrenia*, for 'mind', intending the term to refer to a failure of reliable associations between perception, thoughts and feeling. But these differing terms didn't improve ideas about how to *treat* people awash in a sea of delusions and hallucinations.

How did the flourishing of German mind sciences that saw Alzheimer, Kraepelin and Bleuler transform the understanding of mental well-being give way, by the 1930s, to the Nazified, inhuman psychiatry that saw people murdered in gas chambers for manifesting mental distress? Bleuler's idea of madness as a 'splitting from reality' is perhaps the best way of understanding Nazi ideology – as a splitting away from civilisation, from compassion.

A salient cause must surely include the cult of heredity prevalent then in Europe, which the US also succumbed to in those same years. After a landmark Supreme Court ruling in the 1920s, American eugenics programmes saw the sterilisation of 70,000 people who had been deemed mentally subnormal. The vast majority of these were poor and socially isolated Black women. Of this American eugenics programme Leo Kanner, a Ukrainian-American psychiatrist, now famous for his development of the idea of infantile autism, wrote, 'Shall we psychiatrists take our cue from the Nazi Gestapo?' In 1942 Kanner wrote an article in the *American Journal of Psychiatry* arguing against the euthanasia of the 'feebleminded', citing the evidence of an assistant garbage collector he knew who was 'sober, conscientious and industrious' – he and many people like him, Kanner said, were an integral part of society, and contributed to it. The contrary argument was published in parallel by a neurologist,

Foster Kennedy, who believed that the US should not shrink from such euthanasia. An accompanying editorial sided with Kennedy, adding that parents who resisted the killing of their children were perhaps themselves mentally unwell. In the past, psychiatry has so often got its priorities so very badly wrong that it takes quite extraordinary faith to assume that our current models and practitioners have everything right.

This was the environment in which lobotomy became a routine procedure to render people with distressing chronic psychosis more pliable, and less distressed. Lobotomies involved having sharp implements inserted up through the roof of the eye sockets, severing the connections between the frontal lobes and the rest of the brain, cutting someone off from the most reflective and socially aware part of themselves. More women than men were subjected to this procedure. Its inventor was a Portuguese neurosurgeon, António Egas Moniz (who had hands so gouty he confessed to asking assistants to perform any fine surgical work), who was inspired to try lobotomy in humans by reading about experimental operations performed on laboratory chimpanzees that had rendered them calm and biddable. It was 1935, and the fascist tide was rising across Europe and the US – where his new procedure was taken up with enthusiasm. Four years later Moniz was shot multiple times by a disaffected patient, but survived. In 1949 he was given a Nobel prize – a decision for which the Nobel Foundation has received much criticism. One year later lobotomy was banned in the Soviet Union – the first country to do so.

It's now known that the evangelists of lobotomy (in the US, Walter Freeman and James Watts) were cavalier in their approach to such life-altering surgery, and didn't follow up their patients properly. The British neurosurgeon Henry Marsh has written of encountering numerous patients over the course of his career who had been lobotomised, then abandoned to the back wards of asylums. Even by 1948, the year before Moniz received his prize, lobotomy was slammed in an official report by a 'Group for the Advancement of Psychiatry' who put forward evidence that victims seemed to have 'lost their souls', and that they had become 'shallow and show no depth of feeling'.

Through the later 1950s the advent of major tranquillisers such as chlorpromazine – more effective and more reversible – made the practice of lobotomy obsolete, perhaps because there were other, less gruesome ways of rendering distressed, agitated people more docile. As in the days of Haslam, there was little thought (or hope) of a true cure.

Before hospitals, before psychiatrists, remote communities have always found their own ways of dealing with extreme mental distress. Dramatic shock therapies are common in these histories. In her book *Healing Threads,* the historian Mary Beith summarises some shock traditions of my own country, Scotland. Of the traditional mental health remedies of the Highlands and Islands she wrote, 'By involving the patient in an artificially created drama, the unofficial healer was probably trying to present the abstract, unknowable force of the disease in concrete terms, and by holding up, as it were, a mirror to reality, allowing the patient to come to grips with something more tangible.' She describes an ancient exposure therapy for acute anxiety as being held down on a blacksmith's anvil while the blacksmith swings the hammer at the patient's head, only to deflect the blow at the last second – a provocation not too dissimilar from the 'flooding' therapy of modern psychology. In the church of St Fillans by Loch Earn, 'lunatics' were restrained inside a large hollow stone overnight with a church bell over their heads, given only a covering of hay. At Loch Mo Nàire in north Sutherland, near where I spent a couple of years working as a GP, patients were stripped naked and immersed at sunrise. 'As this was being done coins were thrown into the water,' Beith explains. 'The patients were then pulled out, dressed in silence and walked sunwise around the loch's edge. Then they had to walk away without once turning their heads, until they were out of sight of the water before the sun rose.' The reputation of the loch's healing powers was such that pilgrims continued to arrive even into the 1930s. Further west, 'lunatics' were taken on a journey to a holy isle in Loch Maree to drink water from a particular well. The Welsh naturalist Thomas Pennant went there in 1772 and wrote of its 'power unspeakable in cases of lunacy'.

Nearer to urban centres, in the early twentieth century, there was a vogue for 'shocking' psychotic patients with overdoses of insulin. Their blood sugar would crash to a level so low it was barely compatible with life, then they would be resurrected with infusions of glucose. For some years this treatment was promoted as having transformative results. But then it was shown that it was not the insulin that made the difference, but the intimate and caring attention that, by medical necessity, was being shown to the patients obliged to undergo such a dangerous ordeal. In 1958 the British psychiatrist Harold Bourne said of it that 'Insulin coma treatment may come to be remembered as the first application of psychological healing for schizophrenics in the mass, and its achievement as an inadvertent one – the supply to persons hitherto considered impervious to it, of daily, devoted, personal care.' Insulin or bleeding, a sunrise dip or a voyage to a holy island, a night with your head in a bell, or being mock-attacked by a blacksmith's hammer. Though I might wish them more effective, I'm grateful for the drugs and therapies of today.

The average person spends over twenty years of their lives asleep, and over six years dreaming. 'The death of each day's life, sore labour's bath,' according to Macbeth, in a passage in which he hears voices – 'Balm of hurt minds, great nature's second course, Chief nourisher in life's feast'. Of all possible states of mind, the transitions, perceptions and distortions of dream life seem closest to those experienced in schizophrenia. Many people experience hallucinations in the transition between sleep and wakefulness: this 'hypnogogic' phase can be delicious precisely because it is transitory. It would be difficult to live in such a fluid and unreliable state of mind. The power to hear unseen voices and communicate with beings who aren't present is something that in many cultures is revered, and not uncommon – the ability to unpick the fabric of reality may be a quintessential aspect of our humanity. Psychosis is a difficult subject because it forces us to think about the nature of reality, and the nature of perception – the nature of ourselves.

Delusions are widespread, e.g. that microchips can be put inside vaccinations, or that the world was created in six days. What counts as a psychotic delusion is mostly cultural – we don't think it odd to believe in God, but would think someone delusional who claimed to *be* a god. Studies suggest that among Black people auditory hallucinations that are *not* schizophrenic in nature are more than twice as common as they are among white people, and four times as common as they are among south Asian people. But at the same time, minority ethnic groups in a majority white culture report more paranoid thoughts, almost certainly because of the traumatising effects of accumulated experiences of racism. Social and cultural capital is hugely protective of serious mental illness, and being low on any perceived social hierarchy is to be more at risk of psychosis. One theory proposes that second-generation immigrants are more vulnerable to mental ill-health because what could be perceived as their great strength – the capacity to bridge two cultures – can also become perceived as a weakness: finding it difficult to belong wholly to either.

In terms of triggers, impossible social demands have been proposed to be influential in bringing on psychosis – so called 'double bind' situations in which it's impossible to win between irreconcilable demands. If the situation requiring action or a decision persists and no escape route is available, a psychotic reaction is said to become more likely. Environment and nutrition matter: babies born during the Dutch 'hongerwinter', in which famine was imposed by the German occupying army, had double the schizophrenia risk in adulthood of those born in more plentiful times. Genetics matter: there's a small village in Dagestan, northern Caucasus, of only 3,000 members, which has a 5 per cent lifetime risk of schizophrenia – the highest in the world* – while the Hutterites of South Dakota (all 35,000 of whom are descended from 90 known ancestors) have the lowest risk known, just 0.1 per cent. Much effort in the West has gone into trying to identify those children and adolescents who may go on to develop schizophrenia, so that they can be supported with early and preventative support from child and adolescent psychiatry specialists. But recent research suggests that children who have been under the care of psychiatry for *any* reason, such as mood, eating disorders, self-harm or behavioural problems, have a higher risk of developing psychosis in adulthood. It's possible that a predisposition to psychosis might manifest early as distress affecting almost any realm of the mind.

In *Surviving Schizophrenia* (1982), E. Fuller Torrey, whose sister suffered from psychosis, pushed back against the oversimplification of mental distress, and in particular the idea that complex mental states such as psychosis can be traced

---

* The Palau islands in Micronesia also have a high rate, at 2.5 per cent of the population.

to a single cause. 'Like cancer, it probably has more than one cause,' Torrey wrote. 'Thus, though we speak of schizophrenia and cancer in the singular, we really understand them as being in the plural; there are probably several kinds of schizophrenia of the brain just as there are several kinds of cancer of the brain.' The same has been argued of manic depression, that there may be as many 'types' of bipolar illness as there are people who experience it. And as many autisms. And as many kinds of anxiety. And as many kinds of depression.

The morning clinic had just finished, the last patient had left, and I was beginning to go through my paperwork when the telephone rang. It was Jenna, one of the receptionists, and she wanted to know if I'd take a call from a patient. 'It's Helena,' she said. 'She's been admitted. I think she's phoning from one of the psychiatric wards.'

'Put her through,' I said. I put the paperwork aside, sat up straight, then paused for a moment, taking a breath.

A click, a beep, and then Helena's voice: 'Is that you Dr Francis? Oh, good – now listen: how many realms of mind are there? I remember that night I saw God. It was when had a choice to take a picture, I chose not to, and it was a starry night, that night I saw the UFO, light like a snowflake, a plasma snowflake …'

I'd known Helena for five or six years, a woman in her late thirties who lived with her parents at the far end of my practice area. Twenty years earlier she'd left home to go to art school in another part of the country – at her home I'd seen photographs of her taken at that time: vivacious, wearing bright clothes, hair dyed green and beaming into the camera. When I'd seen her the week before, she was thin and drawn, her black hair, just beginning to grey, had been matted, and she was wearing an old navy duffle coat with some toggles missing. Her mother had brought her in because she'd been kicking over bins again – usually a sign that her mood was going high. At times like this she believed that to hide litter where it couldn't be seen was to fail in our basic duty to accept life in all its imperfections.

What happened at art school only Helena knew, but over the two years that she stayed there she'd gradually fallen out of the orbit of her classmates and the coursework, and into an orbit of her own, involving long tramps to music festivals, sleeping rough on golf courses and in ditches. She was following summonses that no one else could hear. One day she turned up back at her parents' door, having walked 200 miles, apparently without sleeping.

'... like when Superman 2 dissolves into a 2D being, God, was a she, and a 2D entity so she could go through, and it was the correct image of her, in the projection of her, when I get my ashes put in a tube, and I put it there, in London, and put it there, with the guardians of time. Do you think intuition is real? Sometimes it makes people ill, sometimes not, and the more you put up connections, the more you see, and the more you open up your third eye, whereas normally when I'm high I don't need the third eye, if they close down my third eye I won't be able to see the next life ...'

The days, weeks and years since that first time coming home had been a cyclical journey between the loftiest heights of human feeling, when she'd feel elated and awe-struck at the beauty and intricacy of life, and the cold, dark depths of feeling withdrawn, low in mood and despairing of her future. The best times were when she was on her way up: life seemed more engaging, fascinating, alluring and seductive. The patent office must receive many communications from such people in the early throes of a state of mind like this, convinced they have developed an invention that will save all humanity. Obligations and promises, increasingly impossible to deliver, start to pile up.

' ... I can't believe I saw that, above the cathedral, there was the equilateral triangle, the size of two buses but the thickness of a plasma screen, three primary colours inside it, that's why I know it was intelligent life, analysing the structure of my mechanical energy. I put a book on my lap and was about to take a picture, and then it was gone ...'

I listened, giving myself up to the power of Helena's flowing ideas, the pressure of her speech. There was something beautiful yet frightening about the torrent of it; I listened as if privy to a dream.

'... And then she was safe, and now she was a safe encryption of me, in me, I'm glad I didn't take a picture, because it was awe-inspiring, and when I was young all I wanted was to see God ...'

Another long-time patient of mine, Brian, also experiences such episodes, though they are more occasional than Helena's. On his housing estate there was a drug-dealing family that most people in the community know to avoid. They were dangerous – the kind of people who would break someone's legs to make a point, or have a young lad sent to prison purely to smuggle drugs packed into his rectum. During Brian's most dangerous flights of elation he became convinced that he could take that family of drug dealers on, and it was then that his mother would call me. He could communicate with the police without radios, he would say, and if he really needed to get away from a violent situation he could just spread his arms and fly. He also became convinced of his ability to drive like a Formula 1 champion. Why would you worry about breaking the law, when you know you can outdrive any pursuit car? The last time this happened, he crashed at the first junction.

There were home visits to be done, so with reluctance, I told Helena that I was going to have to break off the phone call. Her monologue flowed on regardless, as I warned her once, then again, and then again, before I had to put the phone back down on the receiver. I was glad that she was calling from the safety of the ward, rather than on one of her epic walks.

A few weeks later I saw her at home, more settled in the mind but more sluggish too: a regime of intramuscular injections of strong antipsychotics had begun to take effect. 'Do you remember you called me from the ward?' I asked her.

'Did I? What did I say?'

'You wanted to tell me about a vision you saw, something you'd seen in the sky over the cathedral,' I said.

She gave a wry smile, and a short, smoker's bark of a laugh. 'Oh, Dr Francis, you know better than to listen to a word I say when I'm in that state.'

A notorious puzzle in the study of psychosis and schizophrenia is why outcomes in the West are so disappointing, and outcomes in the global south relatively so much better. The West's comparative atomisation of family networks, the valorisation of the individual over the collective, and its veneration of productive, industrious states of mind and denigration of the converse have all been blamed. It has been pointed out that in poorer countries kinship networks of support may be stronger, and a society with greater tolerance of mystical, transformed states of mind can more readily accept that those states are temporary, and curable. 'The suggestive power of magical-mystic explanations of mental illness and of traditional healing practices may not cure schizophrenia,' says my *Textbook of Cultural Psychiatry*, 'but is likely to lower the barriers to spontaneous recovery and reintegration in the community.' If you view madness as a disease of the brain you gain an objective framework for science to work with, but you also lose the chance of finding something redemptive in the horror of your experience. You may close off the possibility that the experience might be integrated into a meaningful story. The psychotherapist Carl Jung said of this distinction,

> Hitherto we thought that the insane patient revealed nothing to us by his symptoms save the senseless products of his disordered cerebral cells; but that was academic wisdom reeking of the study. When we penetrate into the human secrets of our patients, we recognise mental disease to be an unusual reaction to emotional problems which are in no way foreign to ourselves, and the delusion discloses the psychological system upon which it is based.

Ronald Laing's bizarre bestseller *The Politics of Experience and the Bird of Paradise* hints at this reframing of psychotic experiences. Laing was one of the high priests of the antipsychiatry movement of the 1960s and 1970s, which sought to question the underlying assumptions of prevalent models of mental illness (though he rejected the label 'antipsychiatry'). He argued that madness is a sane response to insane circumstances.

His methods have been largely discredited, and did not lead noticeably to better outcomes for schizophrenia; he was ultimately struck off the medical register. But his insights have value, still. The novelist Hilary Mantel was an admirer of Laing's writings, and once invited me to attend a London seminar she was leading to discuss the book he wrote with his colleague Aaron Esterson: *Sanity, Madness and the Family*. The book was first published in 1964, and Mantel had not long written a new foreword for an academic edition. It describes eleven case studies of women diagnosed as schizophrenic. 'These women are my drowned sisters,' Mantel said as she opened the meeting, 'and with these seminars I am trying to bring them back to the surface.' *Sanity, Madness and the Family* should be thought of as a book about being human, Mantel explained in her foreword, 'about how we cherish and abase each other, how we try to protect each other and sometimes damage each other in the process: about the mechanisms of love and fear, and the individual's gallant, persistent, striving towards a healing that may, to those outside the process, seem like a disintegration.'

A niece and a nephew of one of the women represented in the book were both present at the seminar, and it became apparent that their family's story, as recounted by Laing and Esterson, had been substantially and materially altered for the purposes of the book. A mother described by Laing and Esterson as 'frigid and manipulative' was, said her relative, warm and loving. Other discrepancies emerged over the course of the seminar: relationships described as pivotal in the development of the mental illness were felt by the family to be not entirely as they were represented.

That Laing and Esterson altered the stories of their book may diminish its value as reportage, but I could see that it did not diminish the book's value for Mantel. She was less interested in Laing's work as *science*, than she was interested in the case histories as ways of understanding the numerous impressions, memories, impulses, instincts, embarrassments, ambitions, regrets, loves, desires and humiliations of being human.

'Laing and Esterson did not deny the reality of madness itself,' Mantel wrote of Laing and Esterson's book. 'As clinicians they had seen patients who seemed broken by suffering. But they asked whether the actions and words of these particular patients added up to madness, and if they did, whether it meant anything to delimit that madness as a clinical entity and give it the label of "schizophrenia".' Mental health diagnoses are always constructs, built by consensus, and as such they evolve – homosexuality was notoriously considered a mental disorder until a narrow vote among the American Psychiatric Association in 1973 eliminated it from the *DSM*, and in the American antebellum South, 'drapetomania' was a pejorative diagnosis given to enslaved people who repeatedly attempted to escape bondage. For Mantel, the bizarre behaviours of schizophrenia are 'like the thrashing and clawing of a person who is drowning. They are ineffective and terrifying to behold. They are purposive but look random and wild. They may be counter-productive. But to call them "mad" is a distraction from what is really going on.'

The former psychiatric nurse and novelist Nathan Filer has written extensively about his time working with people suffering from schizophrenia. His book *The Heartland* reproduces long case histories of people who have experienced psychosis, and Filer is careful to note that everything about mental illness remains contested, up to and including the term 'mental illness'. He writes that he first chose to call his book about schizophrenia *The Heartland* because 'it's a condition that defines the discipline' of psychiatry, but at the same time he wonders whether 'the whole concept of the diagnosis has outlasted its usefulness (if it was ever useful) and should be rebuilt from scratch or abandoned entirely.'

One of Filer's most moving case histories is 'Erica', a journalist who developed schizophrenia, the principal feature of which was a paranoid psychosis so profound that she believed she was Britain's most wanted criminal, going so far as to drink bleach to escape conviction. Filer meets her seventeen years after her diagnosis, and describes how she still gets hints of that psychosis returning. 'You know when you kind of sniff something in the air?' Erica tells Filer. 'It's like that. Like just getting a whiff of something. Except it's sniffing a thought.'

'What we call psychosis can also be a response to extreme stress or trauma,' Filer explains. 'For many people it might best be understood as a kind of psychological adaptation, a coping strategy gone awry or a form of storytelling carried out within the mind as a response to unbearably painful life events.' That Erica has found a way to live with her paranoid thoughts, and bravely holds them off, Filer finds 'more than a little humbling'.

The schizophrenias are not understood – we don't know what causes them, and we don't know how to treat them. The boundaries of what constitutes 'schizophrenia' are grey and poorly defined, and the condition seems to manifest differently in different cultures, where it might even have better rates of resolution than in our own western culture. Even in the West, between 10 and 20 per cent of people who have an episode of a schizophrenia-like psychosis will have only one, and it will never return (social factors such as your ability to hold down a job are good predictors). The drugs we use blunt the most prominent, distressing symptoms, and they save lives, but they also come with onerous and dangerous side effects. During the preparations for *DSM-5* it became apparent that the American Psychiatric Association was seeking to broaden the criteria for schizophrenia diagnosis still further, and include a 'psychosis risk syndrome' or even 'attenuated psychotic symptoms' as a milder form of the category. But 'schizophrenia' itself is already so poorly understood that the value of adding this milder version to the *DSM* smacks of overconfidence. If we don't have any tests or effective treatments for the most severe manifestations of psychosis, and we don't have good therapies that reliably prevent them from progressing, the value of identifying 'psychosis risk' is questionable.

'The literature on schizophrenia accumulated over the past century is extensive and suggests at least the outlines of what we don't yet know,' wrote Allen Frances in a critique of the latest *DSM*. 'In contrast, "psychosis risk" is a relative newcomer whose properties remain quite unknown. We don't know how best to define it, can't diagnose it accurately, don't know how to treat it, don't know if treating it has any lasting value, and don't know the extent of its harmful unintended consequences if it were to be made official.' The first principle of medicine is 'Do no harm'; we know now that the simple act of labelling without fully understanding the consequences can do a great deal of harm. Why, then, do we continue to do it?

One of the most powerful accounts I know of describing this kind of mild, or attenuated, psychotic episode is by the late Scottish poet John Burnside, whose memoir *I Put A Spell On You* touches on his time in a Cambridge psychiatric ward. Burnside knew that he had had some kind of breakdown, but many years later was still uncertain what had happened in the days before his admission, and how he got there. 'I knew something had happened to me, and I knew it was intrinsic to who I was, but I didn't believe I was "mentally ill",' he wrote. On the ward he began a friendship with one of the other patients, 'Cathy', who by contrast he describes as a 'classic' schizophrenic, with textbook 'first-rank' symptoms: delusions that her spleen had been removed and her soul with it, and that the TV on the ward communicated secret messages only to her from an orbiting cosmonaut. With *I Put A Spell On You* Burnside is reaching back into his memory and putting together a redemptive, even triumphant interpretation of the way his mind went awry, giving it a new and powerful story. 'I didn't even think I was *mad*,' he wrote. 'Though the word was never used, and it took me years to apply it to the condition that I have been managing all my life, I can see now that I was suffering from a spike in the usual apophenia: the extreme tendency to find elaborate patterns and significance in everything.'

To be able to find elaborate patterns and significance in everything, and then be able to articulate them with language in a way that's both elegant and beautiful, is a great poetic gift. Burnside seems to be suggesting that his tendency towards psychosis, if that is what it was, arose from the same source as his extraordinary art.

11

A TENDER PLACE IN THE MIND:
ON HURTS, SCARS AND ADDICTIONS

Alcohol doesn't console, it doesn't fill up anyone's
psychological gaps, all it replaces is the lack of God.

Marguerite Duras

On the mantlepiece was a photograph taken by a professional, in a happier time. Laura is wearing a pink dress with
a bow around the waist, head tipped back, holding a flute of
fizz. A handsome man in a grey suit stands at her side. 'That
was twenty years ago,' she told me, when she noticed me
looking; 'with my husband. A better time.' Alcohol can act
as a strange, unreliable preservative, keeping the skin youth-
ful even as it stiffens the liver and shrivels the brain. Her face
is puffier now – a nutritious diet is low on her priorities – but
her eyes have the same dancing levity as they had then. She
is still slim, though her liver and the fluid accumulation in her
abdomen has given her an incongruous swollen belly. Slightly
jaundiced, she winces when I press gently. Close up I notice
that her hair is unwashed and smells it, and her teeth are
brown with neglect.

There's a two-litre bottle of cider by the sofa, and next
to it her Jack Russell terrier Sam, who watches me warily
throughout the examination. Laura's brother Simon stands

uneasily by the doorway, perhaps wondering if I'll scold him for supplying her with the alcohol that's clearly killing her. The room is small – he backs out into the corridor to make room when I stand up from my sofa examination. This was a grand house once, the mansion of a merchant, but has been broken up into small flats. It was once among fields, but is now surrounded by 1950s council housing. The wide corridors have been boarded over to maximise rentable space, so that to locate her apartment it's necessary to negotiate a narrow, plywood labyrinth.

I've been here several times before, for crises of varying magnitude. Laura has always refused to go to hospital, leaving me and my colleagues with a conundrum as to how best to manage her binges, withdrawals and pain – damage to the pancreas caused by alcohol has made Laura vulnerable to attacks of agony accompanied by vomiting. She's aware that refusing hospital is risky, but she doesn't trust her brother to look after Sam, and so she stays put. There are legions of patients out there who have problems severe enough to justify hospital, but who are kept at home at their own request.

We agree on a regime of rehydration, alcohol limitation, pain relief, antinausea medication, and I promise to visit again the following day. She tells me again about the photograph: it was taken at a friend's wedding, just a few days before her husband was killed in a road accident by a drunk driver. Laura was pregnant at the time, and shortly after losing her husband she had a miscarriage. 'I have a good reason to drink,' she sometimes says. 'I have the *best* reason to drink.'

Laura's predisposition to epilepsy has been worsened by the swings of alcohol in her bloodstream. Sam is more than just a loyal and loving terrier – he's a clairvoyant rescue dog, able to warn Laura when she is on the verge of having a seizure. When I first met her she was on a regular prescription of anticonvulsant medications but she didn't like the side effects – they made her feel sluggish and weak. On occasion Sam would act strangely: he would jump onto her lap and start yapping, seemingly without provocation. He would put his paws up on her chest, as if trying to push her down onto the sofa or the bed. Her seizures always followed this odd behaviour, and she realised that Sam was giving her a warning – he knew when a fit was coming on. Now, whenever Sam begins to yap like that, she lies down in such a way that she will have less chance of being injured in the throes of a convulsion. 'I couldn't live without my Sam,' she said. 'When he goes, I go.'

Among the many patients I know with alcohol dependency Laura's drinking is unusually overt; for others the drinking is more secretive – sherry hidden in the bookcase, whisky in the garden shed. I knew a traffic warden once who would punctuate his patrol of the streets with visits to public toilets, where he'd lock a cubicle and gulp a few mouthfuls of vodka.

For some it's a routine blood test that alerts me to damaging levels of drinking – alcohol makes red blood cells baggy and swollen, and irritates the normal function of the liver. The call to discuss such blood test results can be a delicate matter – I've had phones slammed down on me for even making a gentle enquiry about alcohol – but most people are genuinely surprised to hear that their drinking has slid into the range where the body and blood are beginning to protest. I raise the alcohol question in part to ask whether there might be any support or specialist referral I can offer, and on occasion a conversation develops in which it becomes clear that drinking is a form of self-medication for a problem that might be more usefully or helpfully addressed.

I had a mentor once, a consultant physician, who had

worked in Scotland's Outer Hebrides where there are strong religious and cultural taboos against drinking alcohol on Sundays. 'The alcoholics there rarely got cirrhosis of the liver,' he told me. 'Sunday was a day of rest for the liver too, and one day a week off the booze was usually enough for it to recover.' Instead of liver disease they'd present with numbness and tingling of the hands and feet, from alcohol poisoning to the nerves (nerves can't regenerate in the same way as liver cells). I had another mentor who worked with miners. 'They'd come out of the pit at the end of the day, straight across the road to a pub with a great long bar,' he told me; 'and every miner knew exactly where along that bar was his place, and at his place several pints would be lined up ready for him. They'd drink eight a day, at least, before going home to their families.' For many of those miners, he went on, drinking was a habit rather than an addiction. 'When they got cirrhosis I'd tell them, "This is because of alcohol, you're drinking too much" – and they would just stop, there and then, no problem.' A unit of alcohol is one small pub measure of spirits, and my mentor told me that in liver clinic he met people who'd get through about a hundred units a week. 'But the psychiatrists, in their clinics, that's a different story,' he said. 'Over there you'll meet people who drink a hundred units *a day.*'

When still very young, perhaps too young, I saw a documentary about addiction. Two scenes have stayed with me through the subsequent decades. In the first, a young man is describing the first time he took crack cocaine. He is a recovered addict, rueful and contrite, but in his eyes there is something wistful, yearning, as he recalls his loss of innocence, almost as if it was an expulsion from Eden. He says that taking crack was like having an orgasm in every nerve of his body – a feeling that he'll forever recall as kind of bliss.

The second image is a neuroscience lab in which a rat has had a probe inserted into what the viewer is told is the reward centre of its brain. By pushing on a lever the rat can stimulate itself electrically, and so it does – again and again, shunning food, or sleep, or water, until it dies.

Through the 1950s and 1960s a Louisianan psychiatrist called Robert Heath supervised a series of deeply unethical experiments in which silver electrodes were implanted across the brains of people with epilepsy, narcolepsy, schizophrenia and, in one widely-publicised case, a gay man who had been ordered to undergo conversion therapy by a court. It was later revealed that Heath was part funded by the CIA. His experiments were poorly designed, and little new was revealed either in terms of how the brain functions or how mental illness might be treated. But he did show how fear and rage can both be evoked by stimulating the same area of the brain (the amygdala). One anonymised subject wore his elaborate electrical stimulation kit while working as a nightclub entertainer, and would repeatedly stimulate an electrode that made him feel as if he were on the verge of orgasm. Another would neglect that button in favour of frantically pressing on one that gave rise instead to a half-grasped memory – an experience that wasn't pleasurable, but irritating. 'The frequent self-stimulations', Heath wrote, 'were an endeavour to bring this elusive memory into clear focus.' Making that electric current run deep in his brain was both an addiction and a compulsion for him. Yearning for a lost and irretrievable past was for him more addictive and compelling than summoning present bliss.

In the specialist field of addiction studies there are broadly two schools of thought which overlap even as they sometimes contradict and fall out with one another. In one camp is the conviction that addiction is a disease, probably genetic, with identifiable brain differences that render someone defenceless against addictive substances, and that one day we'll find targeted individual medications or treatments that will eliminate it. In the other camp are those with the conviction that addiction is always behavioural and environmental, and that it's through social interventions, education, restrictions of access to drugs and alcohol, and diminishing social inequalities that addictions can be defeated. There's plenty of evidence for elements of both. Being a victim of violence or neglect can influence the way certain genes are turned 'on' and 'off', further influencing the development of the brain and changing the way it responds to stress and to cravings, just as can poor nutrition and poor sleep quality. And the reverse is also true: your genetic inheritance influences your behaviour, making you more or less likely to risk falling into addiction.

Many people I care for are suffering the consequences of years of addiction to alcohol, nicotine or street drugs. Addiction is an illness, but my work also shows me daily examples of the individual ways people find to survive it. Any day at all, in almost any clinic, addiction stories surface into conversation, because of the damage drugs and alcohol inflict on the body, and because of the harm they inflict on relationships. These conversations may have their origin in a desperate desire to get an addiction under control, but equally they can arise in passing conversation about family and upbringing, about asthma or blood pressure, about liver tests or finances. In the emergency department rather than the clinic those presentations become more urgent, dramatic and life-threatening, showing how pervasively alcohol and drug use are woven into the fabric of our lives. Were addictive substances to suddenly disappear everywhere, overnight, it sometimes feels as if there would be little left for doctors and nurses to do. Some notes from a single night on call in emergency medicine:

A 51 yr old woman came in cold and staring, brain full of metastatic lung cancer from her lifetime habit of sixty cigarettes a day, and with a dreamy, faraway look in her eyes. She died the following morning.

A 39 yr old man, yellow with end-stage jaundice caught from dirty needles, staring mad, emaciated with stick-like bones. Babbling all night with a ferocious glaring insanity in his eyes, brain aswim in alcoholic delirium.

A 33 yr old woman, with hepatitis, and on methadone, her fourteen-month old baby suckling at her breast. Both mother and child with vomiting and diarrhoea. She lay in a stained Gucci sweatshirt, the beautiful, scabies-infested baby dozing peacefully at her side.

A 30 yr old man, a drug dealer, jumped out of a five storey building to escape the police. Yelling abuse at the two doctors and three nurses it took to attend to his broken ankles.

A 20 yr old man high on cocaine, with a broken wrist, being held down by two policemen. I tried to sedate him and treat him, but he wouldn't let me, so he went back to the cells, screaming in pain, his broken wrist unprotected.

An 85 yr old woman, scant hair matted with thick jelly blood clots, scalp still spurting blood. The police would come back and arrest her in the morning, they said, once she had sobered up. She lay in a back cubicle, happily warbling Abba songs as her blood soaked through the hospital blankets.

A 70 yr old man in a frenzy of agitation, pulling on his IV lines, shouting abuse at the nurses, and swiping at my face. I had to hold him down and inject diazepam into his veins to settle him. The following morning on the ward round he apologised. 'I'm sorry doctor, that was the drink, not me.'

A 35 yr old cocaine and heroin addict, covered in injection site wounds and scabs from her self-harm, wanting her son returned to her from foster care, but too damaged to get herself together to make that happen. Urgently needing to find an alternative way to make herself feel good.

The word 'addict' didn't come into common usage in English until the twentieth century; it comes from the Latin *addictus*, and refers to the idea of delivering yourself over to something, yielding, betraying or selling. But it also has the sense, in Latin, of a devotion or consecration, a sacrifice and abandonment. For some psychoanalysts drug use is best understood as a late-life substitute for a mother's milk. So many sacrifices and abandonments, yieldings and betrayals – all trying to fill an absence.

There are tablets from Sumeria dating to 4000 BCE that make reference to the use of opium; Chinese histories touching on the use of cannabis go back to the origins of writing. Every culture has its ways of inducing altered states of mind, and anthropologists have found that the very few that don't use drugs have evolved elaborate rituals of fasting or sleep deprivation instead. We all need to escape our minds sometimes, somehow. In those Middle Eastern countries without a tradition of alcohol use there are millions of people addicted instead to *khat*, a mild stimulant leaf that's chewed as a panacea for pain, as an aphrodisiac, to help focus in work and at prayer. Drugs are in every society, and in every society it's usually only for a small proportion of people that use becomes problematic.

When patients come to my clinic for help with drug use I explore what their life might be like without it, and whether they're prepared for whatever demons might emerge when they get clean or sober. Some people are unable to keep their drug use within safe limits, and the only way to manage their addiction is to find an alternative less damaging preoccupation or compulsion to occupy the same central place in their lives. Around a third of people who have been neglected or traumatised in childhood develop substance addictions in adulthood, and for those people drugs can be understood as an attempt at self-medication gone awry. Blunting, numbing or even intensifying your feelings can be a means of survival, or of making you feel that life is more valuable.

There is a vast literature on addiction, and a variety of theories as to how it takes root in the mind. There are models that examine our individual vulnerability, our social and environmental surroundings, our personal and intergenerational trauma, our propensity to relapse, and models that focus on the addiction potential of different drugs. One theory emphasises the addict's longing to diminish pain, another the addict's desire for pleasure. Some theories emphasise instead addiction as a heightening of the cravings that drive our need for the basics of perpetuating life: food, drink and sex (known to psychologists as 'incentive salience'). Another view proposes that much addiction behaviour is embedded through the same mechanisms that establish habits ('stimulus response learning'), while yet another theory proposes addiction as the result of poor impulse control and disinhibition.

The field is also divided as to whether 'true' addiction studies should stick with psychoactive substances, or whether addictive behaviours also count. In my own medical practice I've never seen much value in making the distinction: it's clear that sex addiction or video-game addiction can sometimes be as harmful to someone's relationships and livelihood as a drug or alcohol habit, though some specialists wouldn't consider them 'proper' addictions. Gambling *does* tend to make the grade, and I've seen gambling addiction bankrupt families (a weekend binge of most drugs ends in the loss of your dignity and health, but a weekend binge of gambling can finish with the loss of your home). People can become paradoxically addicted to abusive relationships, because they confirm something about the world that doesn't challenge the preconceptions they have built about their own self-worth. They can become addicted to ruminating on things gone wrong, because they're afraid that without that circling negativity they won't be able to get anything right. They can get addicted to shallow relationships, because deeper relationships challenge and threaten their idea of who they are, and who they might become. Whether my patient is grappling with harmful drug use or disruptive behaviours, therapeutic communities such as Alcoholics Anonymous can replace one need with another more supportive one – some of the most effective programmes I've encountered have an element of faith at their core, and build new relationships of care.

All of us are obliged now to connect digitally, and it's common to see people with a different kind of behavioural dependency: young people strung out with Internet anxiety, sleepless with digital overload, who are having difficulty knowing what's real, what's virtual and what their life would be without the Internet. My advice? It has never been more important to find out.

Passing a pub one night I heard a packed crowd singing the Amy Winehouse song about rehab. Winehouse's biography hints at a talent so immense that she lost her boundaries; her fans couldn't or wouldn't see her vulnerability. An occupational hazard of performing seems to be that the dreams and desires of others get projected onto you, and the suicide rate among celebrities suggests that some kinds of fame are more of a curse than they are a reward. The popularity of Amy Winehouse's song about refusing rehab – and its singalong refrain of 'No, no, no' – suggests that among the millions of her fans there are many who needed Winehouse to be a rebel – the chanting chorus asks her to go on embracing addiction so that they didn't have to. Her death set her into a pantheon of numerous other artists and performers who have become totems of the desire of others, that 'it's better to burn brightly and briefly through life than to slowly fade'.

For those for whom addiction becomes a problem, some substance or activity starts by filling a small space in the self that feels empty, but then grows, and grows, until it starts to push out aspects of life that we need in order to live well. It's hard to dig out an addiction; for many the excavation is too wounding and leaves the self vulnerable, weakened and in pain. The open wound that's left behind may need to be treated with gentleness, distraction, medications, in order that it might heal over. For some people it will remain a perennially tender place in the mind, vulnerable to being reopened. But as time goes by it's possible to learn ways of protecting that wound, toughening it up into a hardy and resilient scar – a process that can take years. Whether it's church or faith groups, communities that offer mentors who have been there before you, a relationship with an individual counsellor or a network of friendships, everyone needs to find alternative ways to feel good, secure and protected while giving up an addiction, building in layers of protection over the wound while that tender place has the chance to heal. It's important to develop your sensitivity as to when those layers of protection you've built up over it are getting too thin, because that means that relapse is becoming a risk. To be able to retreat into a more comforting or supportive space until that vulnerability passes is often what's needed.

Mental illness can often be understood as a form of self-expression and self-healing that has gone awry, as much as it can be a surrender. 'Orexia' means desire, or appetite, and so 'anorexia' is the negation of desire and appetite. 'Bulimia' means 'ox-hunger' – a ravenous, insatiable ingestion that carries within its name the flavour of disgust. Eating is one of the most reliable ways we humans have of making ourselves feel good, but some kinds of eating can veer into the territory of addiction – a binge satisfies the same kinds of urges as a fix or an alcoholic session, and a purge of vomiting or with laxatives can feel like a catharsis or climax. Someone who has learned to distrust or close themselves off from the body and its feelings can, through binge eating, experience comfort as well as a series of sensations strong enough to break through the barriers of self-protection they've built up.

Anorexia is often mysterious in its origins: some people become addicted to the airy, light-headed feeling they experience when they're starving; for others its roots seem to go deep into ideas learned in childhood of nourishment, and ambiguity over whether food is good. Or it can be about controlling the boundaries of the self, or it can be a disguised form of self-harm. I'm often struck by how many adolescents who self-starve show a surface indifference to whether they live or die, as if at core they've lost a sense of themselves as someone *worth* feeding.* 'You are someone worth nourishing, you are someone worth caring for,' is the affirmation implicit and sometimes explicit in those conversations I have with young people suffering from an eating disorder.

Teasing apart these different strands and motivations for self-starving or for binging/purging, it becomes clear that the care of eating disorders overlaps with the care of addictions. It requires its own specialised, experienced teams, as well as a great deal of time. Hospital psychiatric services are so often diminished it's not unusual for an eating disorders team to refuse all referrals until a patient's problem becomes life-threatening. The opportunity to intervene early is lost,

---

* I wrote about anorexia in *Shapeshifters* (2018), 'The Enchantment of Control'.

and a perverse incentive is created for those with anorexia to lose even *more* weight before they can be seen by someone with the resources to help them deal with the problem.

Just as eating disorders have some overlap with addictions, so they also overlap with self-harm. When I qualified as a doctor in 1999 the proportion of the UK population who at some time in their life deliberately cut or harmed themselves was around one in forty (2.4 per cent). Young women were most at risk: the figure for those between the ages of sixteen and twenty-four at that time was around one in fifteen.* Just fourteen years later the general population risk had become one in fifteen, and for young women one in *five*. What was driving this huge increase in the number of people who scratch or harm themselves?

Self-harming behaviour is contagious – if you know of someone who does it you're more likely to 'catch' doing it yourself. Your social media use is relevant too: while it offers a supportive network for some, it offers shame, bullying and new self-harm ideas to others – and those who post about their self-harm are more likely to go on to die by suicide. It's not just contagious, it can be competitive: there are communities who compare their scars or bruises or emaciation online. Most of the people I meet who cut are adolescents with exaggerated feelings of low self-esteem, and a haunting disgust or disdain for the self – feelings that have to be put aside, resolved or transcended, even temporarily, for effective recovery to take place. A terrifying new development is the rise of self-harm influencers: people for whom demonstrating their unhappiness online has become a paradoxical source of validation, affirmation, and income. Much self-harm is addictive in the sense that it brings on a feeling

---

* I wrote about deliberate self-harm in *Adventures in Human Being* (2015): 'Punched, Cut and Crucified'.

of separation or distance from intense emotions that is experienced as a reprieve, even a reward. And it is compulsive, in that for many people the cutting relieves an intense anxiety. In a study called 'Self-Harm: Cutting the Bad Out of Me', researcher Jennifer Harris quotes a woman who said of her cutting, 'I really would like to stop self-harming but feel I can't because I am addicted to it. I couldn't live without the release it gives me. The buzz you get from it. If I could find a way of coping without harming myself, it would be fantastic.'

The body produces its own painkilling opiate endorphins when we self-mutilate in this way, inducing the same kind of dissociation that can help survivors of trauma get through – a distanced, dreamlike, unreal state of mind which can in its most extreme manifestations veer into catatonia. And just as the hit of heroin can be prevented by taking an opiate-blocker drug such as naltrexone, so the same opiate blockers can take away the relief that self-harmers feel when they cut. Blocking the effect makes the patient *feel worse* temporarily, because they're not able to separate any longer from their intense anxiety (or, in a traumatised person, the trauma memory), but in the right circumstances those blockers can be an important part of treatment, and of learning less devastating ways of dealing with psychological pain. There is also a powerful symbolism in the shedding of blood, which in itself is a relief. Eating disorders and self-harm have traditionally been separated in terms of how they are framed in diagnostic tables, and in how they are managed, but that separation belies how entangled the roots of both may be, and how close both are to addiction. Another of Harris's correspondents wrote, 'When I started to emerge from my anorexia, I needed some other way of dealing with the pain and hurt, so I started cutting instead. It is a way of gaining temporary relief. As the blood flows down the sink, so does the anger and the anguish.' Harris concluded, 'Purging the self is the act of self-purification. Many of the women who self-harm also engage in purging their bodies of food (we now call this bulimia), and, as a result, many become anorexic.'

Self-harm behaviour among teen boys takes a different form – experimentation with drugs, getting into scraps, dangerous driving – and often ends up being dealt with by the police rather than health services. Self-harm is far more visible to medical staff when there's a need for wound closure, dressings, sutures. The *British Journal of General Practice* once published an anonymous letter from a patient who regularly cut themselves, thanking their own GP for compassionate care. Their behaviour had exposed them over the years to a great deal of insensitive treatment by doctors and nurses, who couldn't understand why they didn't just stop harming themselves rather than troubling their already overstretched departments. 'Both psychiatric liaison teams and some A&E staff can be cold and indifferent as a deterrent, wrongly fearing if they are "nice" this will lead to further visits,' the patient wrote in, while praising their GP for offering treatment without judgement. 'Staff in general practice can make a significant contribution to the care of someone who self-harms frequently. This applies to the receptionists who triage appointments to phlebotomists who do not need to comment when they see a mass of scars. Compassionate care is fundamental and mental health services can lose this.' The patient concluded with gratitude to their practice, and their GP. Acknowledging that self-cutting could look like an addiction, a habit or a 'default setting', the writer wanted to remind clinicians that it was a way of coping with extreme distress.

Sex is among the most powerful drives that affect us as mammals, and much social conditioning is concerned with suppressing or blunting the expression of desire for it. It's a common misperception that our well-developed human frontal lobes are concerned solely with abstract and complex thought; they're also heavily occupied with preventing us from doing things. Among doctors the phrase 'he's a bit frontal' is a euphemism for someone who is disinhibited, who says and does whatever they wish no matter the consequence, as if their frontal lobes are not working properly, not managing to maintain socially appropriate behaviour and responses. In adolescents, the parts of the frontal lobe concerned with playing out scenarios and determining social consequences of actions are not yet fully developed, bringing on the kind of risk-taking that fuels self-harm and addiction. Much of our neural function is dedicated to suppressing urges; what happens when that suppression fails?

Everything in the brain is connected, and damage to parts of the temporal lobes can bring on a comparable syndrome of disinhibition. Klüver-Bucy Syndrome is named for Heinrich Klüver and Paul Bucy, two scientists who in the 1930s observed the effect of temporal lobe brain damage on monkeys. In humans, Klüver-Bucy syndrome manifests as a high sex drive that swerves into socially inappropriate or lewd behaviour, as well as binge-eating, binge-drinking, smoking, and a regression to the kind of orality that babies pass through – assessing objects by licking them or putting them in the mouth. Deep within the temporal lobes are the amygdalae, generators of fear and of anger, and so people with this syndrome sometimes show a bizarre absence of both – they feel calm and unruffled whatever the circumstance, while feeling addicted to sex, and exploring the world with their mouths.

The final piece of writing Oliver Sacks published before his death in 2015 was an essay about Klüver-Bucy syndrome in which he described his role as an expert witness in a trial of a man, 'Walter B', with temporal lobe epilepsy, who had surgery to remove the parts of his brain that were sparking his seizures. Removing those parts of his brain helped his epilepsy, but left him with a ravenous appetite and an insatiable libido. Sacks describes how an addiction, even when purely neuropathological in origin, progresses from a socially disruptive nuisance that threatens relationships, into frank criminality. Having exhausted his wife with his constant demands for sex, Sacks's patient turned first to adult pornography, and (says Sacks, because of online inducements) in time bestial and child pornography. 'Normal control systems have a middle ground and respond in a modulated fashion,' wrote Sacks, 'but Walter's appetitive systems were continually on "go" – there was scarcely any sense of consummation, only the drive for more and more.'

The court ruled that while Walter was not at fault for his physiological compulsions and the brain-state that had given rise to his addictive sexual compulsions, he was at fault for not seeking help. The judge emphasised that his crimes were far from victimless.

Sacks's final essay raises questions of culpability that go to the heart of the distinctions between mind and brain, self and society, and the nature of addiction as an illness. The judge's ruling suggested that personal responsibility endures whatever the origin of an addiction – whether it be in a constitutional tendency, a traumatic childhood, a neurological disorder or simply getting in with the wrong crowd at the wrong time. Millions of pages have been written attempting to find ways of understanding and treating addiction, in part because the origins of our addictions are as many and as complicated as we are ourselves.

Pauline seemed to have found her way through. I got to know her when she reached her mid-fifties, and found it difficult to reconcile the neat, professional businesswoman, the owner of a couple of bars in the city, with the one described in the notes of twenty or thirty years earlier. Her parents had come to London from the West Indies in the 1960s, and she told me she had married too young to get away from them. Her new husband turned out to be a drinker, and he was prone to violent outbursts of rage. To cope, Pauline drank too, including throughout her pregnancy with Diana, her daughter. Being soaked in alcohol while still in the womb had caused Diana some mild learning difficulties, but she'd also been diagnosed in subsequent decades with ADHD, depression, anxiety, and one psychiatrist had suggested that she had an emotionally unstable personality disorder. All these different traits and states of mind might have had their origins in the alcohol with which she was bathed in the womb thirty years ago, or in the chaotic home circumstances of her early life. Recently, Diana had asked me if I could refer her for an autism assessment because, she said, she couldn't make sense of social nuance, couldn't read people, and couldn't cope with the stress of figuring out the intentions of others – yet another potential consequence of alcohol exposure in the womb, as well as a characteristic feature of autism. After a brief liaison with a man who left no forwarding address Diana had a baby now, Sophie. When not caring for Sophie, Diana spent much of her time playing computer games – she described herself as 'addicted' to the online world – but she didn't drink.

Such a chain of addiction: after years of struggling to live independently, becoming a mother had pushed Diana back into needing the support of her own mother, and she and Pauline had moved in together. 'It's safer that way,' Pauline said. 'You should have seen the place she was living in – I couldn't leave my daughter and granddaughter there.' Pauline had signed up as a peer mentor with a local community alcohol action group, giving evening talks about her own story and one-to-one support for addicts. She was having one of her bars converted into a bistro, and hoped eventually to do the same with the other ('Alcohol is for making money, not for drinking,' she said). In the long term, she hoped that Diana might be able to hold down steady work in one of the bistros. Pauline wanted to make amends for years of poor parenting, she said. She wanted to build a different kind of life for Sophie, making sure Sophie would have all the opportunities that had been denied Diana. Guilt was part of it, but also the idea that, by supporting and parenting Sophie, Pauline would find solace and take a step towards restitution of what she saw as her own failings as a new mother all those years ago.

The new arrangement seemed ideal, and I was always delighted to see Pauline or Diana, with or without Sophie, in the waiting room. It seemed as if the story of addiction and family trauma was going to have a happy ending. But a stray comment from another patient made me realise that all was not as it seemed. He described his hellish neighbours in the apartment opposite – a mother, daughter and granddaughter, he said – newly moved in. How he'd see the grandmother stagger in drunk some evenings, struggling even to get her key in the door. The fights he heard through the walls: sometimes it sounded as if furniture was being overturned. The baby's cries that went unattended, the curtains closed until late in the day. 'Terrible to hear that,' the neighbour told me. 'I don't understand why they can't just pull themselves together.'

12

THE MANY DIMENSIONS OF BEING: ON NEURODIVERSITY, AUTISM AND ADHD

These children have come into the world with innate inability to form the usual, biologically provided affective contact with people, just as other children come into the world with innate physical or intellectual handicaps.

Leo Kanner, 'Autistic Disturbances of Affective Contact' (1943)

Neat beige trouser suit, gold studs in her ears, a blouse with a floppy bow at her throat, Nicola presented me with a report from a clinical psychologist in the commercial sector that gave her diagnosis along the top line as 'executive dysfunction'. 'I've always struggled with numbers,' she began. 'I get them the wrong way around, I could never divide a restaurant bill among friends, I could never calculate what wages I should be getting, or what I owe in tax. A friend told me I have dyscalculia, and an occupational therapist I saw once told me I have dyspraxia, because I'm all thumbs.' From time to time she went through phases of binging on food, then purging with laxatives, and running to burn off calories. 'When things are bad I drink too much, but not this time – this time I've got my drinking under control.'

The overriding sense she wanted to explore with me was why she felt so anxious much of the time, and why she felt so low. 'I've definitely been traumatised in my life,' she went on. 'There must be a name for what's wrong with me.' She lived alone, as she'd never found it possible to get on with other people. 'I don't get them,' she said, 'or rather, they don't get me.' I asked her whether she'd say she'd had a happy childhood, and she paused for a moment. 'No, I couldn't say that,' she said. 'Classic only child, of parents who probably loved me, but certainly didn't show it, and they couldn't stand one another.'

'Are they still alive?'

'My mother is,' she said, 'though failing now. And I can't stand that she expects me to be there for her now, when she was so rarely there for me when I was small.'

Her conversation was difficult to follow – it jumped from subject to subject without alighting for long at any one theme, memory or concern. 'I was in the Air Force, you know,' she said at one point, 'but my face didn't fit. Then I worked for the Tax Office, but it didn't fit there either. I can never seem to figure out what others expect of me.' A diagnosis of ADHD was mooted, but a trial of stimulant treatment didn't help her, and the strategies outlined by the psychologist didn't make sense. Old referral letters in the medical notes pointed to a pattern of repeated crisis, followed by referral to psychiatry or to the mental health team, by which time the crisis had passed and she didn't go, or the response came back, 'No enduring mental health diagnosis'. For years she'd been on a low dose of antidepressant medication.

Mood low, alcohol, binging and purging, anxiety and attention problems, poor social skills, dyspraxia and dyscalculia, a neglected, possibly traumatic childhood – I mentioned to her that it would be possible to home in on any one of these and offer a psychiatric diagnosis based solely on that, if she were to find any of them helpful. But at the same time each of those labels would not be expansive enough to describe all her difficulties. I tentatively sounded her out for her reflections on the observation that each of us is a melange of traits, characteristics, hopes, memories, experiences, ambitions and desires, and that a single label can never define our complexity.

'What do you know about neurodiversity,' I said; 'about the idea of dyslexia, attention deficit disorder, autism – different ways of thinking about how the brain works in different people?' She looked down into her lap, at her fingers fiddling with the clasp on her handbag.

'Autism', she replied. 'Yes, could we talk about that?'

The first *DSM* in 1952 described autism as a purely childhood condition: 'schizophrenic reaction, childhood type' – a characterisation of autism as pure pathology, linking it to psychosis in a way that today is utterly unthinkable. The Ukrainian-American psychiatrist Leo Kanner had first drawn attention to autism with his 1943 paper 'Autistic Disturbances of Affective Contact' in the journal *Nervous Child*. 'Since 1938 there have come to our attention a number of children whose condition differs so markedly and uniquely from anything reported so far, that each case merits – and, I hope, will eventually receive – a detailed consideration of its fascinating peculiarities,' he wrote. This 'infantile autism' was a rare, debilitating disorder of social and emotional connection. 'He was happiest when left alone,' wrote Kanner of one of his patients, 'almost never cried to go with his mother, did not seem to notice his father's homecomings, and was indifferent to visiting relatives.' Kanner also noticed that many of the children he studied had family members 'strongly preoccupied with abstractions of a scientific, literary or artistic nature, and limited in genuine interest in people'; Kanner's observation that a spectrum of autistic traits may be inherited and run in families thus goes right back to the earliest writings on the subject.

By 1980 the *DSM-III* included 'infantile autism' among the grouping 'pervasive developmental disorders', listing its features as 'resistance to change' together with 'pervasive lack of responsiveness to people.' Though the diagnostic criteria have broadened and the bar to diagnosis has lowered tremendously since then, the hallmarks of autism remain the same: social and communication difficulties, and restricted, repetitive interests.

One of my holiday jobs when home from medical school was as a nursing auxiliary in a male ward for the long-term care of people with learning disabilities. There were many autistic people being cared for on those wards, their autism just one element among other mental and physical problems. I remember one man, David, who had foetal alcohol syndrome; *his* restricted and repetitive interests manifested as an obsessive fascination for jazz. His father, who had visited promptly every Tuesday for many decades, brought David vinyl LPs, which he would play on a turntable in the day room, wearing headphones, an expression of bliss on his face. Another, Robert, had the profound intellectual disability and limb abnormalities of Cornelia de Lange syndrome; *his* repetitive behaviour was to chew on his forearm, which had to be protected with elaborate strapping to prevent the skin from breaking down. Another resident, George, was in his fifties but had the intellectual development typically seen in a child of three; no single cause for his disability had been identified, and his autism manifested as profound social anxiety that would overwhelm him several times a day. When it came on he would stop suddenly, with a stricken, frozen expression on his face; his eyes would flicker around the room as his limbs began to shake and his bowels loosen. He had to be gently encouraged towards the bathroom without touch, because physical contact was unendurable for him, and made the crisis worse.

It was 1993, and the prevalent diagnostic manual was a revised version of the third *DSM* (the *DSM III-R*). It described autism as an impairment in 'reciprocal social interaction' and 'communication and imaginative activity', with 'markedly restricted repertoire of activities and interests', and set it within an entirely new class of diagnoses called 'pervasive developmental disorders'. 'Some of the least handicapped may eventually reach a stage in which they can become passively involved in other children's games or physical play,' it noted, by way of describing the severity of social difficulties. These more mildly affected children (adults were not mentioned) might 'include other children as "mechanical aids" in their own stereotyped activities'. Autism was then believed to affect around 0.03 per cent of the population, with around four times more boys affected than girls.

Only a year later the *DSM-IV* would reframe the diagnosis entirely, setting the scene for one of the most remarkable revolutions in the way mental disorders have been understood over the course of my career: the utter transformation of autism from that of a rare neurodevelopmental disorder, characterised by profound social and mental dysfunction, to a ubiquitous spectrum of enduring traits which, when concentrated in one individual, can be appreciated simply as an alternative, or diverse, way of being human.

A philosophy of mind based on disease is self-fulfilling, and will see disease everywhere. A philosophy of mind based on diversity will by contrast see ecology and flow, dynamism and evolution, supporting the possibility of change, and of greater ease. Biodiversity, ethnic diversity, cultural diversity: diversity is widely acknowledged to be a good thing, and its application to understanding ways of being, feeling and healing has been illuminating. The term 'neurodiversity' was coined in the 1998 by the sociologist Judy Singer, and has flourished in part because it makes intuitive sense as a concept, and in part because many people with traits characterised as autistic have claimed it as a less stigmatising, polarising and medicalising way of understanding their lives.

The idea of neurodiversity has flourished together with the related concept that as human beings we exhibit a spectrum of traits. The 'spectrum' is now as well-established as the nineteenth-century concept of a 'constellation' of symptoms – the recognition that a series of different medical problems can be seen in clusters that point to a single cause. It's a concept first applied to autism in 1979 by the psychiatrist Lorna Wing, whose own daughter was autistic. Two years later Wing introduced the term 'Asperger's syndrome' into the language of English-speaking psychiatry, as a form of autism first named for the Viennese psychiatrist Hans Asperger, who in the 1930s wrote about a group of mostly boys who lacked social skills, but were adept at abstract thinking and often showed remarkable, oddly uneven intellectual profiles, alongside restricted interests and repetitive behaviours (e.g. ordering their toys in neat rows; hand-flapping when overstimulated). Asperger thought that the positive and negative aspects of autism 'are two natural, necessary, interconnected aspects of one well-knit harmonious personality'. He is often said to have been the first to describe the characteristics of such 'high-functioning autism' (as it came to be called). A decade earlier, in the 1920s, the Soviet physician Grunya Sukhareva had already described a very similar set of autistic characteristics among both girls and boys, and has a better claim to priority.

The incorporation of Asperger's syndrome into the *DSM* alongside autism as a kind of high-functioning variant occurred in 1994, a year after my first experience working on the wards caring for David, Robert and George. 'The syndrome is characterised by strengths such as unusually deep, narrow interests,' wrote the autism researcher Simon Baron-Cohen, 'and challenges in social communication and interaction, in people with average IQ or above and no history of language delay'. The distinction between autism with intellectual and language delay, and autism without such delay, remains a profoundly important one which I'll come back to.

For nearly twenty years the term 'Asperger's' flourished in part because it seemed to give a name and an identity to a great many people who felt different but didn't know quite why, and in part because it was considered a less stigmatising diagnosis than autism. Francesca Happé, a professor of cognitive neuroscience at King's College London, was part of the team that reworked autism's definitions for the 2013 manual, in which Asperger's syndrome was abandoned or rather subsumed into the broader category 'autistic spectrum disorders'. Happé described in a recent radio interview how she came under pressure from some activists to retain the category of Asperger's syndrome in the manual. 'Asperger's syndrome doesn't have any stigma,' they wrote to her, 'and autism does, so you must keep Asperger's syndrome' – to which she replied: 'No, no, no no, no no, no. We're going to destigmatise autism.'

Through the early part of the twenty-first century I met many patients who found the term 'Asperger's syndrome' validating, and helpful both in terms of understanding their strengths and finding a community, but since 2018 the name 'Asperger' has fallen into disgrace. That year evidence emerged that Hans Asperger collaborated with Nazi eugenics programmes, and personally signed referral letters recommending children for transfer to a facility where he knew they would be killed. Asperger's complicity with Nazi eugenic murder is at odds with the humanity of some of his writings, and in his defence, apologists for his actions have pointed to his unusually holistic view of autism, out of step with his contemporaries. He proposed that psychiatric care should focus on adjusting the environment around an autistic person, as well as helping them to build coping strategies for survival in a neurotypical world. 'Our therapeutic goal must be to teach the person how to bear their difficulties,' he wrote. 'Not to eliminate them for him, but to train the person to cope with [their] special challenges with special strategies.'

The word 'neurotypical' to describe a non-autistic person is now standard, but was originally tongue-in-cheek. It was a shorthand term first adopted by the writers of *Autism Network International's* newsletter in the 1990s, to turn the tables on medicalising terminology so often used against people with autism. Contemporary culture is replete with metaphors of 'wiring' in the brain, but the brain isn't 'wired' at all, it's a ceaselessly shifting network of dynamic influences – more like a stream or a whirlpool than a circuit board. But the 'neuro' part of 'neurodiversity' and 'neurotypical' remains a convenient shorthand, rather than a statement of fact, even as fewer and fewer people can be considered 'typical'. Mental states don't sort themselves into tidy categories; they're more helpfully thought of as dimensions of being, overlapping and subject to change. Numbers are controversial because they vary depending on who's counting, and precisely what they choose to count, but by any measure there are now far fewer neurotypical people around, and far more who are considered neurodiverse: over the last twenty-five years the prevalence of autism has exploded. Over that period, among people without intellectual or language disability, it has increased between 700 and 800 per cent, with autism now estimated to affect around one in thirty people. The increase in prevalence across the same period among people *with* intellectual and language disability is far lower, at around 20 per cent.

When a mental state is said to affect around 3 per cent of the population, as autism now does, it has moved from being something best understood as a disorder, into the territory of a common manifestation of the ways humans think, feel and exist. Ubiquitous online questionnaires now suggest to people who'd never considered their own traits or tendencies as autistic to think again. I speak from experience: a questionnaire I filled in recently told me to consider seeking specialist referral for autism myself, though I don't feel distressed or held back by any of the personal characteristics that led to the clinically significant score. Distress is subjective, and I'm at ease with the idea that medicalisation of aspects of our humanity is appropriate if and when they cause distress. According to Happé, a global expert in this field, 'we may well already be at a point where there are more neurodivergent self-identifying people than there are neurotypical, [there] certainly are in my family; so once you take autism, ADHD, dyslexia, dyspraxia, all the other ways that you can developmentally be different from the typical, you actually don't get many typical people left. That's going to change society, but not in a bad way.' Governments all around the world are grappling with the implications of this change in terms of how we think about disability and ability, particularly when it comes to workers' rights, and which conditions are compensated for within the benefits system.

As long ago as 1979 Lorna Wing anticipated this shift – she questioned the usefulness of imagining childhood autism as a specific condition, and pointed out that the traits concentrated under the diagnosis of autism were ubiquitous. She argued that autism was not a category of being, but a dimension of being, just as today many autistic people argue that autism is less of a diagnosis than it is an identity. Before she described autism as existing along a 'spectrum', Wing called it a 'continuum', noticing that though all autistic people seemed to benefit from better structure and support in education, each person could also move up and down this continuum depending on context, on strategies they'd learned, on the environment they were in, and in terms of the neurological and social development. Autism would manifest very differently at different ages. In her interview, Happé summarised the latest thinking on this variable expression of autism depending on context:

> We recognise, at least at the behavioural level, and at the genetic level, that autism, like most things, is just on a continuum, so where you put the boundary for diagnosis there's no natural cut point. Nature doesn't tell us: this side is autism, this side isn't autism. And it's complicated, but it's sort of true that if you took the impairment criteria seriously, you might dip in and out of diagnosis, because when you're at school you might be very impaired by your autistic traits, you're made to do things you don't want to do, you're made to be with people you don't want to be with; when you're an adult, you might find the ideal job, where you don't have to do the things you don't like. Social skills aren't particularly important maybe. And there you might not be impaired by autism. And in theory then you would be below the diagnostic threshold.

I've known many autistic people who have become profoundly disabled and distressed by their way of thinking and being; they feel as if something is missing (a deficit), and even if society were more accommodating of their difference, want their experience to be better, and would rather not 'have' autism. And I've known others who see their alternative mode of being as a legitimate alternative to celebrate and be proud of – health means 'wholeness' and their autism feels complete and whole, just as it is.

As a GP I can't take sides in what is becoming a polarised debate. I don't see it as my role to impose distinctions or make any judgements as to when or how or in which circumstances neurodiversity constitutes disability, or should be considered in terms of deficit. Whichever perspective my patient arrives with, the core of my work remains the same: to attempt to ease suffering. I've known children receive a diagnosis of autism only to refute it in adulthood, and request its removal from their records because they've come to the conviction that it simply took them longer to learn how to navigate the social world. For those people, the label no longer helps them make sense of the world, or accurately describes their experience. That doesn't mean it wasn't true at the time, or even that in some contexts it remains true, simply that a diagnosis based on social difficulties necessarily changes with social context.

The concept of 'neurodiversity' has been a game-changing addition to ways of thinking about the mind and brain, even if it's increasingly difficult to define. To realise that different human traits exist at many complicated and overlapping levels, unique for each person, is to find new ways of understanding and empathising with others no matter how their distress is manifest. It's for this reason that the concept of the autistic 'spectrum', which was so helpful when first proposed by Wing, fits less well into the modern landscape of neurodiversity. The flat image it conjures – a spectrum like a fuel gauge or a ladder of traits – is increasingly being replaced by a more complex understanding that autistic traits exist in uneven or 'spiky' profiles in multiple dimensions.

Just as it's becoming clear there are many autisms, not one condition, and that they exist in many interlocking and overlapping spheres, it's also clear that the clinical view of difference isn't enough; it has to be allied to a humanitarian view that sees value and purpose in alternative ways of being, while remaining ready and willing to help when those alternatives cause pain or distress. Temple Grandin, an autistic woman who has written extensively about her autism, prefers to describe it as a handicap rather than a disorder, in that it slows and limits her capacity to engage socially with others. Grandin's sister is significantly dyslexic, but flourishes in her work as an interior designer because her thinking has always been visual rather than verbal. 'I started to think of autistic traits as being on a continuum,' Grandin wrote. 'The more traits you had on both sides [of the family], the more you concentrated the genetics. Having a little bit of the traits gave you an advantage, but if you had too much, you ended up with very severe autism.'

Further reclassifications and reconfigurations of autism are certain to happen as the term continues to become looser, and more deeply woven into the way we think about thinking. If the history of psychiatry tells us anything it's that the frameworks we use now will be mocked as absurdly simplistic within a few years.

Oscar is a man of forty with close-cropped beard, fashionable clothes, a slight squint. He sits down on the chair and I can see him take a moment to appraise me, deciding how much to divulge, and whether he can trust me. I know he has recently started taking stimulants to improve his attention, was on them for a while as a kid, and that he had to fight to get the diagnosis reinstated in adulthood. I suspect he now wants a higher dose. 'So, how did you get on with the tablets?' I ask him.

They're wonderful, he tells me. He has his life back. He's able to concentrate on the good things in life, and forget about the bad things.

'Bad things?'

He explains: the news, stuff that drags you down, makes you feel bad about yourself. Stupid social media, idiotic, pointless, wasteful froth of media bullshit that can clog your life up with trivia if you let it. 'I can leave it all behind now.'

'And sleep?'

He is sleeping well: eight hours solid, no trouble. And getting up feeling rested, with the desire to go to the gym. Before taking the medications he'd never feel like that – he'd feel glum and down and scattered, unable to decide where to put his attention. But the drugs – now, with the drugs ... 'It's only supposed to be eighteen milligrams, but I've got to tell you, I tried a few days at thirty-six – I just doubled them, and it was even better. That's my level,' he says. 'That's what I need. Maybe we can talk about that later,' he adds, then looks away.

I nod. 'Sure,' and I can feel the pressure in the room ease as his anticipation of conflict evaporates – that I'm not going to argue or dispute his own wishes means that he can begin to relax. 'These tablets can affect your blood pressure, your weight, your appetite, your pulse. I'll need to check those,' I say, and he nods.

His weight is down, blood pressure up, pulse up too: all signs that the higher dose is affecting his body. Or is it just our conversation, his anxiety over sitting in the room with an unfamiliar doctor?

'I've got a tolerance for medications,' he tells me – 'I used to be able to drink four big energy drinks a day, no problem. People'd ask me if it didn't give me the jitters, but no' – he shakes his head – 'those drugs, uppers, caffeine, it just doesn't affect me. It's self-medication. That's why I need a stronger prescription.'

'These drugs are known as "controlled drugs",' I say, 'because there are sets of legal rules around how they can be prescribed.' He nods again. 'And so I can't just double the dose. We've got to do it according to a set pattern, and make sure that you're not having any untoward side effects.' He nods.

'Can I ask you a question?' he asks me.

'Sure.'

'You know autism, ADHD, dyslexia – why are they so much on the increase?'

'There are lots of different ideas,' I said. 'What do you think?'

'If you ask me, it's all the toxins in the environment, all those microplastics, all this stuff we put in our bodies. Autism – you never used to hear about that, now it's everywhere. Why is that?'

There are dozens of theories out there as to why we've seen such huge increases in the diagnosis of neurodevelopmental conditions over the last twenty years. The most notorious is that autism is caused by the MMR vaccine, a theory traceable to a 1998 paper in the *Lancet* by Dr Andrew Wakefield, which has been described as 'the most damaging medical hoax of the last 100 years'. Wakefield's paper described a carefully selected series of just twelve children, and it's now known that Richard Barr, an English lawyer, put Wakefield in contact with them. None of the children was from the London area where Wakefield worked; indeed, one was flown in from the United States to take part. Wakefield claimed 'no conflict of interest', but had received more than £50,000 for his expert work on a lawsuit that Barr was putting together, and had filed patents for alternative vaccines. He has since been struck off the medical register, and his fraudulent paper has been withdrawn.

Measles is thought to have killed somewhere around 200 million children over the last century and a half; a similar number of children are likely to have been brain-damaged by it.* Vaccination with MMR slashes the risk of death or brain damage to almost zero. Following the publication of Wakefield's pseudo-research vaccination rates in Europe and North America plummeted; in Ireland alone (population 4.8 million), it was calculated that within just two years the drop in vaccination led to more than a hundred hospitalisations for measles, and three deaths. And millions of dollars have been spent proving that his study was entirely deceitful: MMR is safe, and does not cause autism. The spurious connection may have caught the imagination of the public because it's around the age of fifteen to eighteen months that MMR is usually delivered, which happens to be the age at which many children begin to manifest autistic traits.

It's not just vaccines: other culprits have been proposed: ultra-processed foods, drugs used in pregnancy, early cord clamping after birth, egg products, overstimulation in early childhood, irritation and inflammation of the digestive tract, carbon monoxide, air and water pollution, pesticides, mercury or microplastics. Public health specialists whose life's work is to carefully comb through millions of data points looking for patterns of exposure haven't been able to find *any* environmental factor that increases the rate of autism. There is a tiny effect determined by your parents' age (autism is more likely if both parents are older than average), and there's also thought to be a small effect of premature birth, and some birth complications.

---

* Around one in 3,000 children who contract measles develop the brain damaging syndrome of 'sub-acute sclerosing panencephalitis' – the younger the child is when measles is caught, the higher the risk.

The jury is in: almost all the increase in diagnosis of autism over the last twenty or thirty years has arisen from broadening of the diagnostic criteria, and wider recognition. At the beginning of this rise, in the 1990s, much of the uptick was due to increased recognition of autism among boys and young men. In more recent years there has been a catch-up in diagnoses among girls, as it becomes more widely recognised how autistic traits may manifest differently between genders. There remain enormous disparities among diagnostic rates between young and old – not because autism is more common among the young, but because older generations are still far less likely to come forward to seek diagnosis, and more likely to frame longstanding autistic traits in other ways.

With such patients I think carefully before bringing up the subject of autism: I've seen the diagnosis be profoundly helpful for someone in their twenties, but be received as nonsensical, redundant or irrelevant to someone in their seventies.

The art of diagnosis is the art of pattern recognition, and for decades now researchers have tried, and failed, to seek patterns in mental health symptoms that point back to underlying causes. Manuals of psychiatric diagnosis are still based on elite groups of clinicians getting together every few years – each with thousands of hours of experience at the coalface of human suffering – and putting the experiences of their patients into clusters.

Some patients who experience cycles of mania followed by depressed mood reject seeing their experience in terms of bipolar illness – they see it instead as their lived truth, their dynamic personality. Mood changes are the air they breathe, the fabric of the world *for them*, and they find it unhelpful to think of those cycles as part of a pathology. This ambivalence over whether to pathologise experience extends across many states of mind and ways of being: outside the realm of mental health the same distinction exists among the Deaf community, some of whom see deafness as an impairment, and others who see it as a difference. The textbooks are full of disorders that are simply exaggerated manifestations of human tendencies, e.g. the line at which impulsiveness shades into something that might be called 'impulse control disorder' is blurred, different from person to person and even moment to moment. Behaviour is always a mode of communication: psychologists who cared for children during the Second World War noted that those who had been evacuated away from their families, and forced to live in dormitories among strangers, often became unruly in terms of conduct and impulse control, but that this ostensibly 'poor' behaviour brought them a benefit in terms of adjustments, care and attention. Winnicott was characteristically concise: 'the problem children, because of their nuisance value, had produced a public opinion that would support provision for them which, in fact, catered for their needs.'

The word 'ability' originally meant 'having sufficient power or means', and arose in the early fourteenth century from the Old French *ableté*: 'capable; fitting, suitable; agile, nimble'. Its origin is the Latin *habilem* and *habilis*: 'easily handled, apt'. *Disability* from this definition suggests someone difficult to handle, clumsy, unsuitable, incapable. The first published description of a syndrome of disabling attention deficit was by the Edinburgh physician Alexander Crichton, in 1798: 'it becomes evident at a very early period of life, and has a very bad effect, inasmuch as it renders him incapable of attending with constancy to any one object of education. But it seldom is in so great a degree as totally to impede all instruction; and what is very fortunate, it is generally diminished with age.'

Like autism, ADHD has undergone a transformation in the last thirty years, from a rare disorder thought to affect a small number of children to a ubiquitous aspect of humanity's neurodiversity, with the potential of a label conferring the sense of lifelong disability. In Crichton's city of Edinburgh psychiatric referrals for assessment of adult ADHD recently went from taking up 3 per cent of the total referrals to be assessed by a psychiatrist, to 25 per cent of all referrals, within five years – a phenomenon due to what has been called *metanosis*: becoming aware late in life that one of your personal characteristics might be accorded a clinical diagnosis. The American Center for Disease Control and Prevention recently reported that ADHD was now diagnosed in over a *fifth* of all fourteen-year-old boys and almost a *quarter* of seventeen-year-old boys. There are now 7 million American children with a diagnosis of ADHD, up from 6 million in 2016, and 2 million in the mid-1990s.

A recent study in Iceland found that the country now has the highest rates of ADHD in the world – one in five of *all* adolescent boys are in receipt of a prescription for ADHD, and one in ten adults between eighteen and forty-four. Rather than herald this as an example of welcome improved recognition of a common problem, the Icelandic authors urgently called on their Icelandic colleagues to pull back on this 'overdiagnosis' and 'overtreatment'. The truth is that no society knows what the 'right' level of ADHD among a population should be – there is a core of severely affected people, but the majority are in a grey zone which meets criteria for a diagnosis under some circumstances, but not under others.

As autism is often characterised as a deficit in both social skill and in breadth of interests and behaviours (implied by the phrasing 'narrowed' or 'repetitive'), so ADHD has baked into its very name the idea of 'deficit'. But some adults with ADHD have nevertheless chosen to understand it as a difference with its own compensations or consolations. An ADHD community magazine, *ADDitude*, lists twelve 'super-powers' that people with ADHD might conceivably benefit from, including energy and creativity, acceptance of difference and, paradoxically, hyperfocus. Alongside stock images of happy, smiling families running across meadows and playing science games in a laboratory, the article on twelve superpowers is published alongside another titled 'Seventeen things to love about your ADHD!'

The psychologist William James insisted that 'the fact of voluntarily bringing back a wandering attention, over and over again, is the very root of the judgement, character, and will.' To be constitutionally unable to focus attention can be profoundly disabling. In the West we speak of mindfulness as a practice of being aware of the moment in a state of open attention, without being snagged or tangled in emotion. Many techniques of mindfulness come back to noticing, slowing and experiencing each breath as the basis and the basic rhythm of life. Learning to control the wandering of attention with meditation and mindfulness techniques has been shown to be an effective, drug-free treatment for ADHD. It's often noticed that kids with ADHD are not suited to traditional approaches to classroom learning, in which the children are obliged to stay seated for long periods of the day focused on desk-based tasks. A culture of flickering images, scrolling and short videos feeds acute sensitivity to boredom, which has also been shown to worsen symptoms of ADHD. A recent study found that American teenagers now average around sixty seconds' capacity to focus on a task; office workers average only three minutes.

Amphetamine drugs were first used in the control of hyper-activity by the Rhode Island psychiatrist Charles Bradley in the 1930s. Bradley gave Benzedrine to a group of thirty children who had been characterised as having behavioural problems.

Their teachers reported a remarkable improvement in school performance in around half of them. As with lithium and its effect on mania, the discovery was by accident: Bradley had initially tried Benzedrine as a painkiller for headaches caused by having had air pumped into the ventricles of their brains in order to show up brain structures on X-rays. The headaches didn't improve, but he noted marked improvements in behaviour. He was surprised that stimulants could cause the children to become more attentive and subdued.

> It appears paradoxical that a drug known to be a stimulant should produce subdued behaviour in half of the children. It should be borne in mind, however, that portions of the higher levels of the central nervous system have inhibition as their function, and that stimulation of these portions might indeed produce the clinical picture of reduced activity through increased voluntary control.

More recently evidence has emerged that stimulant treatments seem to work largely through the way they make you *feel*, rather than necessarily improving how you *perform*. When compared with placebo, stimulant drugs tend to provoke greater effort and motivation, but those efforts are of lower quality overall, and any learning achieved under the influence of the medications is poorly maintained. In adulthood it's common to dip in and out of taking medication for ADHD depending on whether you're called upon to do boring repetitive tasks, and in that they still have value: if a task is so easy that performance doesn't matter much, then these drugs will help anyone bear its monotony, and make them feel as if they're doing something worthwhile. People with ADHD feel as if their threshold for loss of focus is lower, and so the drugs feel even more helpful. In terms of academic performance in children the benefits are modest and short-lived.

In a recent interview between the education journalist Paul Tough and the neuroscientist and ADHD expert Francisco Xavier Castellanos, the latter said of stimulant treatment: 'The first dose is almost like a mystical experience, you see this transformation. The behavioural benefits are really sort of stunning, especially in younger kids.' But Castellanos doubts whether the drugs really help these kids learn in the longer term. 'There's a real disconnect between the almost awesome effects on behaviour and the minimal effects on academic achievement or attainment. What bothers me is that the kids do more seatwork – you can see that they've done more problems – but then when you test them a week or two later, their scores barely budge. Or they don't budge at all.' Beyond about a year of treatment, the main effect of using stimulants in children is to stunt their growth. We are asking parents to make a bargain: better behaviour, in exchange for losing an inch or so of height. There's growing concern too that years of treatment with ADHD drugs may substantially increase the risk of subsequently developing Parkinson's disease – a disorder triggered by the depletion of brain dopamine. The acceleration in use of these stimulants for ADHD in adults is so recent that we don't yet have enough data to know whether or not they are safe in the long term. And that's without considering the shorter term negative effects of ADHD drugs that we already know of; pharmaceutical companies list as 'common' or 'very common' the following: 'aggression (or hostility); alopecia; anxiety; appetite decreased; arrhythmias; arthralgia; asthenia; abnormal behaviour' – and that's only the side-effects beginning with 'a'.

As with autism, the explosion in numbers of people diagnosed with ADHD can be seen as a worrying overmedicalisation of an aspect of human difference and variability, or it can be seen as a welcome expansion of acceptance that there are different ways of being. Whether I'm talking with patients who have normal intellectual and language abilities, like Nicola or Oscar, or with patients who have a learning disability, like David, Robert, and George, I find the latter perspective most helpful. But both have an element of truth.

When autism causes distress and suffering, the most helpful interventions have long been known to be social and educational, and there are parallels with ADHD. In my city there's an adult support group with the witty title of Procrastination Station, where people who find it difficult to attend and focus can meet with others who identify with the same difficulty, to share advice and support. Communities matter: the Deaf Way Festival brings together thousands of deaf people who come from all over the world, bringing their different sign languages but united in the experience (and identity) of being deaf. In autistic communities a similar transformation has been affected by initiatives such as Autreat, a festival or gathering of thousands of autistic people who benefit from growing and strengthening their sense of community. Steve Silberman, in his book about neurodiversity, *Neurotribes,* noted that 'the notion that the cure for the most disabling aspects of autism will never be found in a pill, but in supportive communities, is one that parents have been coming to on their own for generations.' In such gatherings an abiding sense of difference, of never fitting in, of feeling alien among groups of others, gives way to a welcome sense of belonging and ease.

Communities of professionals who think about mental health are beginning to realise that the West's twentieth-century focus on individualism has led it to create maps of the mind that have many blind endings. It's possible that the intensely competitive, relentlessly social culture of the modern West is making more and more people feel that if they don't fit into it, they might have a disability. It's a pity that when someone struggles with social interaction, which is something we engage in collectively, our culture currently places all the fault into the individual and labels it as disorder.

For too long mental illness was understood as an aberration of brain function, with too little acknowledgement that our minds exist embedded in relationships of care or neglect, pleasure or suffering, validation or dismissal. Even before birth we are woven into relationships – unborn babies learn the prosody and melody of language, and of familiar voices, through the walls of the womb long before they can distinguish words; we are cared for or neglected long before we are born. Our dependence on caring relationships with others broadens, deepens and becomes more complex as we grow and learn. Much suffering as an adult has its roots in difficulties with approaching, forming and sustaining relationships with others, and with managing and regulating the way we express and experience our emotions.

This matters because autistic traits by definition make interpreting someone's intentions more difficult. Body language, tone of voice and facial expression don't come together so intuitively as to convey a particular emotional state, so it can take more explicit cognitive effort to read between the lines of someone's behaviour. That's exhausting, whether it's making sense of flirting, boasting, or of being threatened. It can be more difficult to tolerate uncertainty when you rely on patterns to make sense of the world. Being expected to read fluently when you're dyslexic, or manipulate numbers when you're dyscalculic, provokes similar levels of anxiety and stress. Finding it difficult to focus your attention whether or not you find a task boring, when work or school obliges you to do just that, is also exhausting – more so when you live immersed in a digital culture explicitly engineered to maximise stimulation and distraction.

When some people realise that their intolerance of uncertainty, or their difficulties interpreting the intentions of others, or the restlessness of their attention, are part of a constellation of traits shared with many others, that can be affirming and reassuring. The difficulties themselves haven't changed, but framed differently they become part of a different story. They take on a life of their own, external to the self, no longer seen as a personal failing but as a personal attribute to be cherished or, where those traits bring only distress, at least understood.

HOPE AND THE UNFRAGILE MIND

He is the best physician who is the most ingenious inspirer of hope.

Samuel Taylor Coleridge

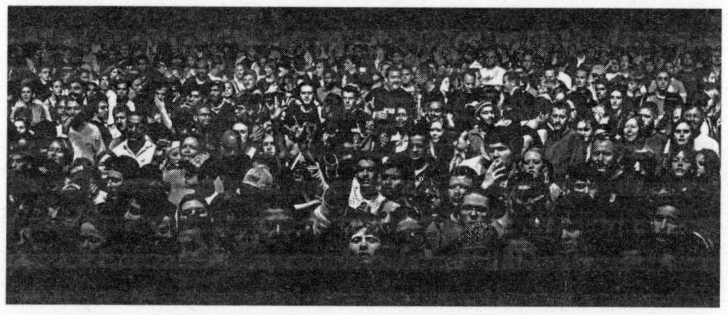

Homo sapiens might have been around for half a million years or so, but our history goes back barely 5,000. The human adventure is only just beginning. Life can be difficult for everyone, and though we cannot undo or avoid the hardships that come with it, we can nudge our reactions, and learn the hard arts of self-compassion and self-awareness. The happiest people I've met have found ways of enduring or making peace with those hardships – no easy task. A scientific approach to suffering began only three or four centuries ago, and is now confirming that our well-being is about more than chemicals or cells – it's about relationships.

The greatest work on the health of the mind to emerge from this earliest science was Robert Burton's *Anatomy of Melancholy*, a sprawling polythesis of discursive hearsay and erudite scholarship, a baroque monument of digressions and circumlocutions, of rumination and personal experience. It's majestic and at the same time majestically unwieldy: its first edition in 1621 ran to more than 900 pages; modern editions are longer still. Keats said it was his favourite book; Samuel Johnson counted it among the best of bedtime reading. Burton concluded with a few words of distilled wisdom that remain as useful for sufferers of mental illness now as they were then: 'Be not solitary, be not idle, SPERATE MISERI CAVETE FELICES [unhappy ones, have hope; happy ones, be cautious].'

Burton called himself 'Democritus Junior', because he was an admirer of the Greek philosopher Democritus, who 2,000 years earlier had been preoccupied with the secrets of human happiness. For Democritus the aim of life was to develop an attitude of cheerful flexibility, confidence and the absence of fear by allowing a diversity of interests and enthusiasms to flourish, honouring and strengthening relationships with others, and taking as much care for the soul as we do for the body. It remains sound advice.

For each of my patients life has a different purpose and meaning, and much of the trick of a happy life lies seems to lie in figuring out what works best *for them* to help bend with life's challenges, rather than be shattered by them. Life is like a flame, in that its heat, crackle and light spring from the raw material of time, creating and consuming moments in the same hot breath. Life is like a river, in its relentless, irresistible flow that can be moulded and diverted but never truly blocked. Life increases in value to the extent that we actively cherish it, believe in it and pursue its possibilities. Life is quantum, atomic, molecular, biochemical, physiological, neural, psychological and emotional, but, standing over all of these, it is social. Relationships rewire our brains, and the habitual thoughts we dwell on change our chemistry. It's natural to long for the reassurance of simple explanations of why we suffer, but if we know anything about the universe, it's that it isn't simple. Its great consolation is that change isn't just possible, it's inevitable.

Life is a balance of energies, good and bad, up and down. It may be difficult to look on its bad aspects, but we can acknowledge them then, like a gardener with her seedlings, tend and strengthen and support those elements that grow towards the good. There hasn't been enough written about the importance of tenderness and attention in the making of a flourishing life. Most of the suffering I see in clinic arises from loss, fear, and from misdirected or thwarted love. Friendships and families, satisfying work, belief in the value and purpose of living – these are the time-honoured ways of building a contented life, and all of them require at least a degree of effort, which should always be balanced with periods of ease. Heaven and hell are right here on earth, and the keys to both lie strewn around us. All the major world philosophies agree on common elements to be aspired to in a life well lived: humility, compassion and having reverence for other lives, and for life itself.

Just as effort and ease should be in balance, so should doubt and belief: uncertainty makes us free to live and learn, it gives us opportunities to change focus and modify our path, in full humility that we'll never know or understand it all. Physicists tell us that nothing is ever pre-determined – uncertainty is baked into the very foundations of the universe. A century ago the polymath J. B. S. Haldane summed up this idea as 'the universe is not only queerer than we suppose, but queerer than we can suppose ... I suspect that there are more things in heaven and earth than are dreamed of, or can be dreamed of, in any philosophy.' It's worth staying humble about how little we really know.

Current diagnostic frameworks of psychiatric diagnosis imply an unjustified degree of certainty; we need to give ourselves the latitude to doubt. Almost forty years ago the psychiatrist Robert Kendell wrote that

> 'schizophrenia' and 'manic-depressive illness', and all our other diagnostic terms, are simply concepts. They are products of the human imagination, and they exist only in the realm of ideas. The only fundamental question we can ask about them, therefore, is whether they are useful concepts, and even that question has to be quali-fied further – useful to whom, and in what context?

We owe it to ourselves to keep on asking that question.

Every doctor or therapist is a bundle of possible selves, and every clinical consultation is different opportunity for something new. Sometimes I'm asked to be a healer, some-times a technician, sometimes a confessor, sometimes a witness, sometimes a scribe, sometimes an arbitrator. The writer and GP Iona Heath wrote to her friend, the art critic John Berger,

> I seem to be groping towards the idea that just by lis-tening and responding gently and thoughtfully I could begin to help my patients to tell slightly different stories; ones which revealed more of their undoubted reserves of courage and endurance in often appalling circum-stances, and stories which would somehow lessen their burden of shame and allow them greater stature and presence.

No two patients' stories are ever the same, but there are

patterns that recur, and the work has shown me that although there are numberless possibilities unfolding in every moment of every life, each person's experience can be influenced and shaped for the better. Psychiatric drugs, though they have side effects, are often helpful and frequently life-saving, but are only a small part of the story. The hope of my profession is that even the most appalling situations can be mitigated in *some* way, however modest, even if it's only to restore a sense of hope, or of being cared for. The best psychiatry is focused on strengths rather than weaknesses.

Mental illness cannot be separated from the social and emotional life of the person who suffers. Diagnosis should always be a process open to revision, and we must learn to hold the labels that we apply to states of mind more lightly and with more flexibility. In recent years much has been written about the need for an utterly new map for making sense of our states of mind, but no new and better paradigm is yet available. There's a move to take away the barriers between diagnoses, and see all mental suffering as existing along different spectrums; another movement suggests classifying disorders by best guesses at what causes them; yet another suggests bringing all diagnostic categories down to the level of neurobiology. The increasing willingness to see childhood trauma and neglect as influential across the long arc of a life is a step towards a kinder, more informed psychiatry. Among clinical psychologists rather than psychiatrists there is enthusiasm to move away from diagnostic categories altogether towards a 'transdiagnostic approach' which focuses on underlying vulnerabilities and poor coping strategies, which may result in very different symptoms between different people. But no alternative is yet sufficiently developed to take over as a new framework.

Maps are not the territory, and we would do well to remember that lists of diagnoses are just *ideas,* not statements of fact, and convey nothing of the subtlety and delicate interplay of strengths and vulnerabilities that make up each individual. States of mind are dimensions of being, not categories of illness. And our current categories of mental ill-health still have their uses in terms of making sense of suffering, offering patients an explanation and a community of others from which to draw support and reassurance, and in suggesting which treatments *might* have the best chance of helping. The ever-increasing complexity of the *DSM* and *ICD* manuals means they are of ever-diminishing usefulness to many clinicians – both too specific and too blunt for research, too clumsy and unwieldy, so sprawling in their categorisations that the edges of what constitutes illness as opposed to health are increasingly difficult to define.

It's a complexity that is driving part of the enormous recent increases in prevalence of mental illness, while at the same time making it seem ever more difficult for people to get the help that they need. The consultant psychiatrist Rebecca Lawrence, in her candid memoir of her own episodic severe mental illness *An Improbable Psychiatrist*, put it like this: 'There is now far more emphasis on talking about mental illness or mental well-being, but sometimes I wonder if the noise of this talk actually makes it harder to hear.' As a culture we have a mania for categorising mild to moderate mental and emotional distress as a necessarily clinical problem – a tendency which is new in our own culture, and not widely shared with other cultures. We now export our approach to psychiatry with as much zeal and enthusiasm as we once exported missionaries. This would be fine if there was no evidence such an approach can cause harm but there's gathering evidence that the wrong labels can do a great deal of damage. Intercultural psychiatrists point out that in many non-western societies low mood, anxiety and delusional states are seen as spiritual or religious problems, not psychiatric ones. By making sense of states of mind through terms that are embedded in community and tradition, they may even have more success at incorporating our crises of mind into the stories of our lives.

Health has been defined as 'the silence of the body', but no one's mental and emotional life is silent, and as we become quicker to pathologise common and even normal experiences we risk burdening otherwise healthy people with the idea that they are deficient or disordered. I've known patients who've been given four or five different diagnoses in their lives, though their core symptoms (and distress) have remained the same. For those patients, labels have been at best a distraction, at worst a travesty of misdirection. When I trained in community medicine I was introduced to pathways and cul-de-sacs of the mind that I'd never encountered in hospital medicine, and began to see how each person has a unique blend of experience, genetics, resilience, character and resources. We speak often now of neurodiversity, but it's as helpful to think that as human beings we possess an abundance of 'psychodiversity'.

The word psychodiversity was coined by the psychologist Michael Apter over twenty years ago, to get over his frustration with psychology's preoccupation with identifying stable 'traits', either positive or negative. 'To be healthy is to be unstable – to be able to move between different kinds of personality to suit the occasion,' he wrote in 2003.

> If biodiversity is necessary to the health of an ecological system, then what we might call 'psychodiversity' is just as important to the health of the individual: it allows them to adapt to ever-changing and relatively unpredictable environments, and also to have a life that is rich with experiential diversity and that allows for the expression of all sides of their personality.

It's a wild world out there; lush, unpredictable, and teeming with ways of being human. The term 'psychodiversity' captures that range, especially if it can be expanded beyond Apter's definition to embrace modes of being that can feel negative as well as positive, as the term 'neurodiversity' does.

Every week I am shown examples of how dynamic our mental well-being can be across the decades of a life, and how current frameworks for making sense of mental illness are too rigid for the reality of our changeable, infinitely adaptable, unfragile minds. Psychiatrists are a little bit like astronomers, trying to understand the patterns within the galaxy of each patient, drawing lines of connection, understanding the way life events have arranged the gravitational pull of their symptoms into constellations. Looking to the future, I wonder what new connections might be drawn between the stars that guide my patients' lives.

The very dynamism of the mind is a perennial source of hope: sometimes the best service a doctor can perform is the reassurance that things *can* and *do* get better – after all, they've personally seen it happen many times before. We are all bundles of possible selves, and it can be helpful to imagine each mind as a dance of time and flow that exists in motion – a perpetually evolving present that is subject to change, indeed *must* change from moment to moment, in all of its uncertainty. That we human beings evolved in the world and were co-created *by* the world, are ourselves an inextricable part of nature as much as any tree or butterfly, is immensely reassuring, and another reason for hope.

The psychiatrist Benji Waterhouse recently summed up the key to human happiness. 'It's really very simple,' he wrote;

> all you need is a healthy birth, secure attachment, happy childhood, minimal or no trauma, high resilience to

stress, loving friends, family and partner, fulfilling work, financial security, manageable targets, eight hours' sleep a night, regular exercise, healthy diet, access to nature, limited use of alcohol, drugs and social media, faith or spirituality, an acceptance of failure and death, an ability to process grief, a naturally positive outlook, maybe a pet, a gratitude journal, plus or minus antidepressants, therapy, and 100 per cent charge on your phone.

Easy, then. Note that Waterhouse didn't mention anything about serotonin levels in the brain, but focused on social, emotional, developmental and attitudinal aspects of life as the building blocks of happiness. It's known that if you have a serious and disabling mental disorder such as schizophrenia, you benefit more from having access to housing, financial security and a community of others than you do from any kind of drug, no matter how innovative or expensive.

The psychologist Mihaly Csikszentmihalyi summed up a lifetime's research into human satisfactions when he concluded, 'People were happiest when they were just talking to one another, when they gardened, knitted or were involved in a hobby; all of these activities require few material resources, but they demand a relatively high investment of psychic energy.' He also noticed that watching TV made people feel less happy or satisfied than other tasks or hobbies, because it placed so few demands on the mind.

I sometimes ask my patients: what brings you strength? Perhaps it is noticing and cherishing beauty in the world around you, even if it's only the flowers in a window box or a face changing into a smile. Perhaps it's remembering the vulnerability of everyone, and realising that most people are only pretending that they have their life under control. Maybe it's working with your hands to make things, tend things, care for things. Pet owners (and particularly,

dog-owners) tend to be happier than average, and so are gardeners, perhaps because the care they give to other kinds
of life returns to them, amplified (vegetable gardeners tend
to be more content than ornamental gardeners). Taking
care of what and how you eat: most people are happiest at
mealtimes spent with others, and for some the key to happiness lies in the preparing and the sharing of food. Being in
green space and among green smells, having leisure – time
to sit in the sun, reflect, and write. To be reminded of the
grandeur of the universe, and your relative insignificance,
can put your troubles back into perspective, whether that's
watching the sun rise in the morning, or finding the time to
notice the sunset. To hear the sound of running water is to
be reminded that everything is flow, and nothing stays the
same for long – as does listening to music, which organises
our scattered thoughts, and channels them into an art and
pleasure that is as transient as it is fulfilling. I had a patient
for whom listening to birdsong in a park or garden was a
reliable, accessible tonic, with its melodies woven of sky, and
flight, and time. Give something back to your community
– people who volunteer are happier than people who don't.
Celebrate with others: joining with hundreds or even thousands at a live concert induces a kind of dissociative joy, a
mood and emotion augmented for being shared. Get active
and use your body however you can: be glad of what it can
do, rather than be shy or embarrassed about what it can't.
Children learn to sing nursery rhymes, clap with others, and
play ring-a-roses, because rhythm and timing and movement
are fundamental to our sense of feeling grounded in our
bodies, part of the world, and at ease. For some, strength
depends on getting away from the demands of children for
some me-time; for others it's helpful to deliberately spend
more time with young children, for whom hope is as natural
as breathing. There are so many ways to expand the circle of

your awareness, even in solitude: reading or rereading great stories, or beautiful poems, or old journals, or mind-blowing science. Think of good things that you've done, and never stop learning. And for those with mental illness that orbits into severe, life-threatening territory sometimes, it's important to find a doctor or therapist they can trust. Continuity of care matters – being able to get a non-urgent appointment to see the *same* doctor – because a fifth, tenth or twentieth conversation with someone about matters of such importance as your state of mind is necessarily deeper and more valuable than the first.

Though we can't change the past, we can always influence the future. Every action we make has the potential to change the world in some small way; those changes may nudge other events, which inspire others, until even a small difference in how you spend a day, hour or minute can influence the unfolding of the world.

For too long psychiatry and psychology have focused on the individual, both in terms of vulnerability and pathology, and in terms of resilience and autonomy. From the 1980s the field of mental health became dominated by ideas of brain cell neurochemistry, and overlooked the reality that our minds are co-created by the relationships that sustain us. We are utterly interdependent with others, and always have been – that was the key to the survival of our distant ancestors, and it's the key to our survival now.

The psychotherapist Victor Frankl observed that happiness can't be *pursued*, that it must *ensue* as a consequence of a life well-lived. Happiness isn't a noun, it's more like verb or even an adverb – it's a way of *doing* or of *being*, rather than a static state of mind. If bodily health is experienced as a silence of symptoms, mental health too is experienced as ease and flow. Modern living offers such a plurality of possibilities and conflicting, competing demands for our attention that it's easy to become scattered and distracted, for the flow of the mind to become turbulent rather than smooth, and this too lies at the heart of some of the consultations I have with people who have lost goals and focus. If the meaning of life *is* meaning, sometimes it's my role to help people to choose among the myriad opportunities of their lives what their focus and purpose could be. Though everyone must find such purpose within themselves, it's a privilege to engage in such conversations every day.

Anxious, traumatised, high, low, deluded, addicted, neurodiverse, we are all vessels for thoughts, feelings and desires that wash through our being, influencing our sense of self and contentment, and in these pages I've sought to set out some ideas to be taken further, to experiment with, to weigh, accept and also reject if better ones come along. The ways we understand the mind are always changing, but the elements of what makes for a happy life remain the same: love and work, community and connection, effort and ease, change and flow. Be not solitary, be not idle; happy ones, be cautious; unhappy ones, have hope.

LIST OF ILLUSTRATIONS

While every effort has been made to contact copyright-holders of illustrations, the author and publishers would be grateful for information about any illustrations where they have been unable to trace them, and would be glad to make amendments in further editions.

THANKS

To my patients, for the trust they place in me, and for the insights they've given me into their many ways of living and being.

To Kay Redfield Jamison, for her magnanimity in allowing me to quote from her work. Adrian Doyle generously permitted me to quote from his letter to his sister, Miranda, about their shared childhood, reproduced in Miranda's *A Book of Untruths* (Faber, 2017). I'm very grateful to all the authors and their publishers cited across the arc of this book; in particular for the eloquence and expertise of Nathan Filer, Lucy Foulkes, Jay Griffiths, Iona Heath, Hope Jahren, Noreen Masud, Iain McGilchrist, Bruce Perry, Maia Szalavitz, Bessel van der Kolk and Benji Waterhouse.

I'm thankful for the kindness, encouragement, erudition and warmth of the late Hilary Mantel and the late John Burnside; Hilary's invitation to join the seminars she was leading on sanity and madness was characteristic of her generosity. I'm very grateful to Sarah Burnside and Robin Robertson for granting permission to quote from John's 'I Put A Spell On You'.

As a teacher, Sophie O'Brien has helped me think differently about fragility and resilience. To my mentors – skilled clinicians and teachers who showed me the ways medicine should be an alliance of science and kindness: among them Alex Connan, Jim Gallagher, Tom Gillingwater, Khazeh Fananapazir, Mike Ferguson, Gordon Findlater, Fanney Kristmundsdottir, Sandy Reid, and Janet Skinner.

To Hayden Lorimer and Hester Parr, extraordinary geographers, for inviting me to join their research into Seasonal Affective Disorder, and to Professors Roy Robertson and Bruce Ritson, for the benefit of their many decades of experience working with addiction. Thanks to Dougal Brown for help with the pictures. I'm indebted to psychiatrists Naida Forbes, Wojtek Wojcik, Kate Womersley, Iain McClure, Lucy Calvert and Neil McNamara for talking to me about the themes of this book, and giving me valuable insights into the challenges and rewards of their specialist work.

To my colleagues in general practice: Will Chambers, Julie Craig, Peter Dorward, Erik Jespersen, Ruth McLean, Kieran Sweeney, Lizzie Wastnedge, Ishbel White and Fiona Wright, for our many shared discussions about this difficult but rewarding profession, exploring how to do the best by our patients.

Profile Books and Wellcome Collection have encouraged and supported me now for over a decade writing books about medicine and culture – 'thanks' doesn't go far enough to acknowledge the debt I owe to Fran Barrie, Penny Daniel, Andrew Franklin, Cecily Gayford, Rebecca Gray and Hannah Ross. Graham Coster copy-edited the manuscript with enthusiasm and alacrity. Thanks too to my agent Jenny Brown for the haggis, as well as the many contracts and connections we've made and strengthened over the years.

Some passages of chapter nine were previously published as a long read in the *Guardian* entitled 'What I have learned from my suicidal patients' in November 2019 – I'm grateful to Clare Longrigg for permitting them to be presented here.

My deepest gratitude of all is for my family.

NOTES

Introduction: Adventures in Thinking, Feeling and Being

p. 1   'You doctors come across …': Munthe, Axel: *The Story of San Michele* (John Murray, 2004).

1. The Box of Delights

p. 7   'There is a great deal …': Eliot, George, *Daniel Deronda* (Penguin, 2012).

2. Constellations of the Mind

p. 23   'Those who first …': Berger, John, *And Our Faces, My Heart, Brief as Photos* (Bloomsbury, 2005).

p. 23   'Other ancient epics describe …': see Sheth, Hitesh C., Gandhi, Zindadil and Vankar, G. K, 'Anxiety disorders in ancient Indian literature', *Indian Journal of Psychiatry* 52(3), July–September 2010, pp. 289–91.

p. 26   'Life is inherently difficult …': Winnicott, Donald, *The Child, the Family and the Outside World* (Penguin, 2021).

p. 27   'My new diagnosis …': Wang, Esmé Weijun, *The Collected Schizophrenias* (Penguin, 2019).

p. 27   'Sometimes I wonder if …': Waterhouse, Benji, *You Don't Have to be Mad to Work Here* (Cape, 2023).

p. 28   'A recent survey …': see *Dispatches*: 'Young, British & Depressed', aired Channel 4, 29 July 2019, 8 p.m. Referenced in https://happiful.com/documentary-reports-mental-health-crisis-amongst-young-people (accessed September 2025).

p. 28   'broadened the net …': Kessler, R. C. and Wang, P. S., 'The Descriptive Epidemiology of Commonly Occurring Mental Disorders in the United States', *Annual Review of Public Health*, vol. 29 (April 2008), p. 115–29.

p. 31 'dry, fatigued, frail …': Estés, Clarissa Pinkola, *Women Who Run With the Wolves* (Picador, 2008).

3. Physicians, Priests and Prophecy

p. 35 'It is the history …': Stevenson, R. L., in a letter to Edmund William Gosse, November 1879.

p. 36 'Keeper of the Royal Rectum': see Porter, Roy, *The Greatest Benefit to Mankind* (Harper Collins, 1997).

p. 38 'Grasping anything trustworthy …': Aristotle, *De Anima*, i 1 402 a5-a11.

p. 38 'Consciousness is a …': Sutherland, N. S. *The International Dictionary of Psychology* (Crossroad, 1995).

p. 41 'The science writer …': on placebos, see my essay on placebos in the *New York Review of Books*, 'What Do You Expect?', 26 June 2025.

p. 43 'over 400 separate categories …': see this cogent article arguing for a shift from *DSM*'s categorical system to a dimensional approach: van Heugten-van der Kloet, D., and van Heugten, T., 'The classification of psychiatric disorders according to *DSM-5* deserves an internationally standardized psychological test battery on symptom level', *Frontiers in Psychology*, 4 August 2015, 6:1108.

p. 45 'sum of all possible …': see Ellenberger, H. F., *Psychiatry from Ancient to Modern Times* (Basic, 1974).

p. 45 'energetic interference often …'; Munthe, Axel, *op. cit.*

p. 45 'Most psychiatric conditions …': Katona, C. and Robertson, M., *Psychiatry at a Glance* (Blackwell, 1995).

p. 47 'Once the impression …': Rosenhan, D. L., 'On being sane in insane places', *Science*, 179 (4070), 19 January 1973, p. 250–8.

p. 47 'In 2017 a homeless man …': Yang, Maya, 'Man arrested in mistaken identity case locked in Hawaii mental health hospital for two years', *Guardian*, 4 August 2021.

p. 48 'All scientific knowledge …': see Ellenberger, *op. cit.*

p. 48 'in the work of science only …': *ibid.*

p. 48 'the more one thinks …': Darwin, Charles, *More Letters of Charles Darwin* (John Murray, 1903).

p. 49 'maybe labels are useful …': letter dated 5 April 2000, quoted in Heath, Iona, *Ways of Healing* (OUP, 2024).

p. 49   'It wasn't important *which* …': see Neighbour, Roger, *The Inner Consultation* (Routledge, 1987).

p. 49   'Understanding what is "wrong" …': Van der Kolk, Bessel, *The Body Keeps the Score* (Penguin, 2014).

p. 50   'The diagnostic exuberance …': Aftab, Awais, 'Conversations in Critical Psychiatry: Allen Frances, MD', *Psychiatric Times*, 23 May 2019, vol. 36, issue 10.

p. 51   'This explicit admission …': see Mezzich, J. E., 'Culturally informing diagnostic systems', in S. Barnow and N. Balkir (eds), *Cultural variations in psychopathology: From research to practice* (Hogrefe, 2013), pp. 137–53.

4. Chemicals to Networks

p. 53   'Despite decades of …': Frank, Jerome and Frank, Julia, *Persuasion and Healing* (Johns Hopkins, 1974).

p. 53   'Dr George Ashcroft had argued …': Eccleston, D. and Ebmeier, K., 'George Warburton Ashcroft' (obituary), *Psychiatrist* 34(7) (2010), p. 307.

p. 54   'the volume of … tripled …': Lockhart, P. and Guthrie, B., 'Trends in primary care antidepressant prescribing 1995–2007: a longitudinal population database analysis', *British Journal of General Practice*, 61 (590), September 2011.

p. 54   'The *DSM* is not …': Hacking, Ian, 'Lost in the Forest: Who Needs the *DSM*?', *London Review of Books*, 8 August 2013.

p. 55   'I strongly believe …', Jamison, Kay Redfield, *An Unquiet Mind* (Picador, 1996).

p. 56   "I succeeded at …': Insel, Thomas – interview with Adam Rogers in *Wired*, 11 May 2017.

p. 57   'Biology never read …': Insel made this remark to *The New York Times* at the time of the publication of *DSM-5*.

p. 59   'In 2017 a Dutch …': Borsboom, Denny, 'A network theory of mental disorders', *World Psychiatry* (2017), 16:5–13.

p. 63   'The great topmost sheet …': Sherrington, Charles, *Man On His Nature* (Cambridge, 1951).

5. Formative Experiences

p. 66   'Infant care, like doctoring …': Winnicott, *op. cit.*

p. 72   'People are complex …' Perry, Bruce and Szalavitz, Maia, *The Boy Who Was Raised As A Dog* (Basic, 2017).

p. 77 'the close relatives …': Berger, John and Mohr, Jean, *A Fortunate Man* (Canongate, 2015).

p. 81 'Exposing a person to …': Perry *op. cit.*

p. 82 'Here is another …': Winnicott, *op. cit.*

6. Living on Red Alert: On Anxiety, Anguish and Fear

p. 88 'fear spread thin': see Crowcroft, Andrew, *The Psychotic* (Pelican, 1967).

p. 91 'The space that occupies …': de Jong, J. and Hinton, D., 'Traumascape', in Bhugra, D. and Bhui, K., *Textbook of Cultural Psychiatry* (Cambridge, 2018).

p. 93 'SmithKline Beecham …': for a fuller discussion of SmithKline Beecham's campaign see Harrington, Anne, *Mind Fixers – Psychiatry's Troubled Search for the Biology of Mental Illness* (Norton, 2019), p. 255.

p. 94 'In the rush …': Foulkes, Lucy, *What Mental Illness Really Is … (and what it isn't)* (Vintage, 2021).

p. 99 'What we call psychosis …': Filer, Nathan, *The Heartland – Finding and Losing Schizophrenia* (Faber, 2019).

p. 100 'I don't like heights …': Shawn, Allen, *Wish I Could Be There: Notes from a Phobic Life* (Viking, 2007).

p. 106 'a great way …': Clare, Tim, 'My life was ruled by panic attacks, so I spent a year tackling my anxiety. This is what I learned …', *Observer*, 22 May 2022.

7. The Worst Already Happened: On Trauma and Personality Disorders

p. 109 'They were shit parents …': Adrian Doyle's epilogue to Doyle, Miranda, *A Book of Untruths* (Faber, 2017).

p. 110 'in the UK one child is …': child deaths due to abuse or neglect: statistics briefing (NSPCC, 2025).

p. 110 'adverse childhood experiences (ACE)': Felitti, Vincent J. *et al.*, 'Relationship of Childhood Abuse and Household Dysfunction to Many of the Leading Causes of Death in Adults', *American Journal of Preventive Medicine*, 14 (1998), pp. 245–8.

p. 111 'overall a fifth of children …': Foulkes, *op. cit.*

p. 112 'In the *ICD* … 6B40': *ICD-11* can be accessed here (September 2025): https://icd.who.int/browse/2025-01/mms/en#2070699808.

Notes

p. 113 'the personality is ...': Janet, P., *L'Evolution de la Personnalité* (Société, 1984).

p. 113 'other expressions of distress ...': Hinton and de Jong, *op. cit.*

p. 113 'Recovery can be expected ...': https://icd.who.int/browse10/2019/en#/F43.1 (accessed September 2025).

p. 115 'even in the bad cases ...': quoted in Kendell, R. E., 'The distinction between personality disorder and mental illness', *British Journal of Psychiatry* 180 (2002), pp. 110–15.

p. 115 'problems in functioning ...': see ICD-11, https://icd.who.int/browse/2025-01/mms/en#941859884 (accessed September 2025).

p. 116 'Certainly, it is commonplace ...'. Kendell, *op. cit.*

p. 117 'There appears to be ...'; van der Kolk, B. D. and van der Hart, O., 'Pierre Janet and the Breakdown of Adaptation in Psychological Trauma', *American Journal of Psychiatry*, 146 (12), December 1989, pp. 1530–40.

p. 118 'The shifts in identity ...': Fidyk, Monika *et al.*, 'Dissociative Identity Disorder: A Comprehensive Review of Etiology, Diagnosis, Neurobiology, and Treatment', *Quality in Sport*, vol. 41, 12 May 2025. p. 60277.

p. 118 'DID develops when ...': Dorahy *et al.*, 'Dissociative Identity Disorder – an empirical overview', *Australian and New Zealand Journal of Psychiatry*, vol. 48(5) (2014), pp. 402–17.

p. 120 'If the shorthand of ...': Masud, Noreen, *A Flat Place* (Hamish Hamilton, 2023).

p. 121 'if patients ... are told ...': van der Kolk, *op. cit.*, p. 289.

p. 125 'the automatisation of ...': Ludwig, A. M., 'The Psychobiological Functions of Dissociation', *American Journal of Clinical Hypnosis*, 26(2) (1983), pp. 93–99.

p. 126 'The idea of self-care ...': Timimi, Sami, *Searching for Normal* (Fern Press, 2025).

p. 128 'By some measures ...': Fedynich, A. L. *et al.*, 'Brief novel therapies for PTSD', *Current Treatment Options in Psychiatry* (6(3) (2019), pp. 179–87, and Fischer, I. C. *et al.*, 'Post-traumatic stress disorder: rethinking diagnosis', *Lancet Psychiatry*, 10(10) (2023), pp. 741–2.

p. 131 'Some studies ...': Perry and Szalavitz, *op. cit.*

p. 132 'thereby living in a new ...': Pinkola Estés, *op. cit.*, p. 391.

8. A Fire Hose of Epiphanies: On Mania and Elation, Wonder and Awe

p. 134 'It seemed as though ...': Beers, Clifford, *A Mind that Found Itself – An Autobiography* (Longmans, Green, 1910).

p. 142 'Ghastly encounters with emptiness ...': see McGilchrist, Iain, *The Matter with Things* (Perspectiva, 2021), p. 291: 'In severe depression many patients report no feelings at all, and in such cases even seeing it as a mood disorder at all presents philosophical problems.'

p. 143 'Four times in her life ...': Woolf, Leonard, *Beginning Again* (Hogarth, 1964).

p. 145 'Lithium's origin story ...': Draaisma, Douwe, 'Lithium: the gripping history of a psychiatric success story', *Nature*, 26 August 2019.

p. 147 'severe psychopathology inhibits creativity ...': Holm-Hadulla, R. M. *et al.*, 'Creativity and Psychopathology: An Interdisciplinary View', *Psychopathology*, 54 (1) (2021), pp. 39–46.

p. 150 'You don't fear life ...': Jahren, Hope, *Lab Girl* (Knopf, 2016), p. 145.

p. 150 'Then I saw my wings ...': Griffiths, Jay, *Tristimania* (Hamish Hamilton, 2017).

p. 151 'When you're high it's ...': Jamison, *op. cit.*, p. 67.

p. 153 'characterised as "arrested fear"': by James Leuba, American psychologist.

p. 154 The Goodall Institute video is here: https://www.youtube.com/watch?v=jjQCZClpaaY.

p. 155 'humble veneration': see Evans, H. M., 'Wonder and the Clinical Encounter', *Theoretical Medicine and Bioethics* 33 (2012), pp. 123–36.

p. 156 'Often after I have gone ...': Carlos Williams, William, 'The Practice', in *Doctor Stories* (New Directions, 1984).

9. Tears Blue, and with a Wounded Heart: On Depression, Melancholia and Suicide

p. 158 'It is wrong to believe ...': Durkheim, Emile, *Suicide: A Study in Sociology* (Routledge, 2002).

p. 160 'It's also perfectly possible ...': a mixed feeling explored in Norman Bradburn, *The Structure of Psychological Wellbeing* (Aline, 1969).

p. 162 'However, all cultures ...': Bhugra, D. and Bhui, K., *Cross-Cultural Psychiatry* (Arnold, 2001). Professor Bhugra went on: 'Prevalence rates for depression have been shown to be consistently higher for women than for men across all cultures ... Some cultures are more likely to present with somatic symptoms or social loneliness or alcoholism, depending upon how culture allows the symptoms to be identified and developed. Some symptoms may be universal, according to the WHO collaborative study of depressive disorders (including sadness, joylessness, hopelessness, anxiety and lack of energy) ... Bereavement can often lead to depression, but mourning and rites related to the death of an individual vary dramatically across cultures.'

p. 166 Posternak, M. A. *et al.*, 'The naturalistic course of unipolar major depression in the absence of somatic therapy', *Journal of Nervous and Mental Diseases* 1294 (2006), pp. 324–9.

p. 167 Cuijpers, P. *et al.*, 'The outcomes of mental health care for depression over time: A meta-regression analysis of response rates in usual care', *Journal of Affective Disorders* 358, August 2024, pp. 89–96.

p. 167 'huge research effort ...' Moncrieff, J. et al. 'The serotonin theory of depression: a systematic umbrella review of the evidence', Molecular Psychiatry 28, 3243–3256 (2023).

p. 167 Mariner, A. S., 'A critical look at professional education in the mental health field', *American Psychologist*, 22(4) (1967), pp. 271–81.

p. 171 Styron, William, *Darkness Visible* (Vintage, 2001).

p. 174 'Military esprit can ...': Durkheim, *op. cit.*

p. 176 Kasai, Y. *et al.*, 'Psychological effects of meditation at a Buddhist monastery in Myanmar', *Journal of Mental Health*, 26:1, (2017), p. 4.

10. Privy to a Dream: On Psychosis, Delusions and Hallucinations

p. 179 'Should delusion come to... .': Wang, *op. cit.*

p. 180 Hearing The Voice website, https://hearingthevoice.org/, accessed September 2025.

p. 180 'Over the course of ...'; King's College London press release, 19 October 2024: https://www.kcl.ac.uk/news/spotlight/the-power-of-digital-avatars-in-psychosis-therapy (accessed September 2025).

p. 182 Haslam, John, *Illustrations of Madness* (Hayden, 1810). Available on archive.org in September 2025.

p. 187 'It would appear that once ...': G. Bateson (ed.), *Perceval's Narrative* (Stanford University Press, 1961), quoted in Laing, R. D., *The Politics of Experience* (Penguin, 1967).

p. 189 'Over the course of ...': see Engstrom, E. J. and Kendler, K. S., 'Emil Kraepelin: Icon and Reality', *American Journal of Psychiatry* 172 (12), September 2015.

p. 190 'Shall we psychiatrists take ...': Joseph, J., 'The 1942 "euthanasia" debate in the American Journal of Psychiatry', *History of Psychiatry*, 16 (62 pt 2), June 2005, pp. 171–9.

p. 191 'hands so gouty ...': Tan, S. Y. and Yip, A., 'António Egas Moniz (1874–1955): Lobotomy pioneer and Nobel laureate', *Singapore Medical Journal* 55(4), 4 April 2014, p. 175–6.

p. 192 'By involving the patient ...': Beith, Mary, *Healing Threads – Traditional Medicines of the Highlands & Islands* (Birlinn, 2018).

p. 193 'Insulin coma treatment ...': Bourne, Harold, 'Insulin Coma In Decline', *American Journal of Psychiatry* 114 (11), May 1958.

p. 194 'among Black people ...': Johns L. C. *et al.*, 'Occurrence of hallucinatory experiences in a community sample and ethnic variations', *British Journal of Psychiatry* 180 (2002), pp. 174–8.

p. 194 'report more paranoid thoughts ...': Bhugra and Bhui, *op. cit.*

p. 199 'The suggestive power of magical ...' *ibid*, p. 225.

p. 200 'Hitherto we thought ...': Jung, C. G., 'The content of the psychoses', In C. G. Jung and C. E. Long (ed.), *Analytical Psychology* (Moffat & Yard, 1916), pp. 312–51.

p. 201 'about how we cherish and abase ...': Laing, R. D. and Esterson, A., *Sanity, Madness and the Family*, with a foreword by Hilary Mantel (Routledge, 2016).

p. 202 'it's a condition that ...' Filer, *op. cit.*

p. 202 'You know when you ...': *ibid*.

p. 203 'between 10 and 20 per cent ...': Rosen, K. and P., 'Predicting Recovery From Schizophrenia: A Retrospective Comparison of Characteristics at Onset of People With Single and Multiple Episodes', *Schizophrenia Bulletin*, vol. 31, issue 3, July 2005, pp. 735–50.

p. 203 'The literature on schizophrenia ...': Frances, Allen, 'The British Psychological Society Condemns DSM-5', *Psychiatric Times*, 26 July 2011.

p. 204 'I didn't even think I was *mad* ...': Burnside, John, *I Put A Spell On You* (Cape, 2014).

11. A Tender Place in the Mind: On Hurts, Scars and Addictions

p. 206 'Alcohol doesn't console ...'; Duras, Marguerite, *Practicalities: Marguerite Duras Speaks to Jérôme Beaujour* (Grove, 1990).

p. 210 'conversion therapy by a court ...': Heath employed a young female sex worker in an attempt to 'convert' the patient to heterosexuality while undergoing brain stimulation. See O'Neal, C.M. *et al.*, 'Dr Robert G. Heath: a controversial figure in the history of deep brain stimulation', *Neurosurgical Focus*, vol. 43, September 2017.

p. 210 'The frequent self-stimulations ...': Heath, R. G., 'Electrical Self-Stimulation of the Brain in Man', *American Journal of Psychiatry* 120, December 1963, pp. 571–7.

p. 219 'I really would like to stop ...': Harris, Jennifer, 'Self-Harm: Cutting the Bad Out of Me', *Quantitative Health Research*, vol. 10, issue 2, March 2000, pp. 164–73.

p. 220 'Staff in general practice ...': Anonymous, 'Long Term Self Harm – a patient perspective', *British Journal of General Practice* 73 (736) (2023).

p. 221 'essay about Klüver-Bucy': Sacks, O., 'Urge', *New York Review of Books*, 24 September 2015.

12. The Many Dimensions of Being: On Neurodiversity, Autism and ADHD

p. 225 'These children have come ...': Kanner, L., 'Autistic disturbances of affective contact', *Nervous Child* 2 (1943), pp. 217–50.

p. 229 The *DSM-IIIR* is available here (accessed September 2025): https://archive.org/details/diagnosticstatis00amer_1/page/34/mode/2up.

p. 230 'It's a concept first ...': Feinstein, A., 'Lorna Wing', in Volkmar, F. R. (ed.), *Encyclopedia of Autism Spectrum Disorders* (Springer, 2013).

p. 230 'Two years later Wing ...': Wing, L., 'Asperger's syndrome: a clinical account', *Psychological Medicine* 11(1) (1981) pp. 115–29.

p. 231 Baron-Cohen, Simon, 'The Truth about Hans Asperger's Nazi Collusion', *Scientific American*, 17 May 2018.

p. 231 *The Autism Curve*, BBC Radio 4, episode 2. Broadcast August 2025.

p. 236 'I started to think …'; Grandin, Temple, quoted in Silberman, Steve, *Neurotribes* (Allen & Unwin, 2015).

p. 238 'the most damaging …': Flaherty, D. K., 'The vaccine-autism connection: a public health crisis caused by unethical medical practices and fraudulent science', *Annals of Pharmacotherapy* 45(10), October 2011, pp. 1302–4.

p. 241 'the problem children …': Winnicott, *op. cit.*

p. 242 'it becomes evident …': Lange, K. W. *et al.*, 'The history of attention deficit hyperactivity disorder', *ADHD Attention Deficit and Hyperactivity Disorders* 2(4), December 2010, pp. 241–55.

p. 242 'there are now 7 million …': Tough, Paul, 'Have We Been Thinking About A.D.H.D. All Wrong?', *New York Times Magazine*, 13 April 2025.

p. 243 'A recent study in Iceland …': Ingimarsson, O. *et al.*, 'High prevalence of treatment with ADHD medicines indicates overdiagnosis of ADHD in Iceland', *Laeknabladid* 110(9), September 2024, pp. 402–10 (Icelandic with abstract in English).

p. 243 'superpowers': This article in *ADDitude* was initially published as 'Positives of ADHD: 12 Amazing Superpowers', but later edited to 'What I Would Never Trade Away', in part in response to differences in opinion within the ADHD community as to whether such language represents 'toxic positivity' and can ultimately prove unhelpful. See https://www.additudemag. com/slideshows/positives-of-adhd/ (accessed September 2025).

p. 243 'Learning to control the wandering …': though its success is limited in younger children. See Lee, Y.-C. *et al.*, 'Effects of Mindfulness-Based Interventions in Children and Adolescents with ADHD: A Systematic Review and Meta-Analysis of Randomized Controlled Trials', *International Journal of Environmental Research and Public Health* 19 (2022), 15198.

p. 243 'shown to worsen symptoms …': Chuxian, X. *et al.*, 'The Separation of Adult ADHD Inattention and Hyperactivity-Impulsivity Symptoms and Their Association with Problematic Short-Video Use: A Structural Equation Modeling Analysis', *Psychology Research and Behavior Management* 18, 1 March 2025, pp. 461–74.

p. 243 'Bradley gave Benzedrine …': Bradley, C., 'The behavior of children receiving benzedrine', *American Journal of Psychiatry* 94 (1937), pp. 577–85.

p. 244 'show up brain structures ...': Lange, K. W. *et al.*, 'The history of attention deficit hyperactivity disorder', *ADHD Attention Deficit and Hyperactivity Disorders* 2 (2010), pp. 241–55.

p. 244 'It appears paradoxical ...': Bradley, *op. cit.*

p. 244 'those efforts are of lower ...': Bowman, E. *et al.*, 'Not so smart? "Smart" drugs increase the level but decrease the quality of cognitive effort', *Science Advances* 9 (2023), eadd4165.

p. 245 'The first dose is almost ...': Tough, *op. cit.*

p. 245 'developing Parkinson's disease ...': Baumeister, A. A., 'Is Attention-Deficit/Hyperactivity Disorder a Risk Syndrome for Parkinson's Disease?', *Harvard Review of Psychiatry* 29(2), 1 March–April 2021, pp. 142–58.

p. 245 'aggression (or hostility) ...' 'British National Formulary, Open Source Version 3.2.34 (464) updated 01 October 2025, accessed 22 October 2025.

Conclusion: Hope and the Unfragile Mind

p. 249 'He is the best ...': Coleridge, Samuel Taylor, *Table Talk and Omniana* (G. Bell, 1884).

p. 250 'Be not solitary ...': Burton, Robert, *The Anatomy of Melancholy* (Penguin, 2023).

p. 251 'the universe is not only ...': Haldane, J. B. S., *Possible Worlds* (Chatto, 1927).

p. 252 '"schizophrenia" and "manic-depressive ..."': Kendell, R. E., 'The major functional psychoses: Are they independent entities or part of a continuum? Philosophical and conceptual issues underlying the debate', in A. Kerr and H. McClelland (eds), *Concepts of Mental Disorder: A Continuing Debate* (Gaskell/Royal College of Psychiatrists, 1991), pp. 1–16.

p. 252 'I seem to be groping ...': Heath, *op. cit.*

p. 253 Holliday, R. *et al*, 'The Evolution of the Classification of Psychiatric Disorders', *Behavioural Sciences* (Basel) 6 (1), March 2016, p. 5.

p. 253 'Among clinical psychologists ...': Dalgliesh, T. *et al.*, 'Transdiagnostic Approaches to Mental Health Problems: Current Status and Future Directions', *Journal of Consulting and Clinical Psychology* 88(3), March 2020, pp. 179–95.

p. 254 'There is now far more ...': Lawrence, Rebecca, *An Improbable Psychiatrst* (Cambridge University Press, 2024), p. 83.

p. 255 'To be healthy …': Apter, Michael, 'On a certain blindness in modern psychology', *Psychologist* 16 (9), September 2003, pp. 474–5.

p. 256 'All you need is …': Waterhouse, *op. cit.*

p. 257 'It's known that …': see 'Changing Psychiatry's Mind', my review of Anne Harrington's *Mind Fixers* in the *New York Review of Books*, 14 January 2021.

p. 257 'People were happiest …': Csikszentmihalyi, Mihalyi, *Flow* (Harper & Row, 1990).

p. 257 'Pet owners … vegetable gardeners …': Jacobs Bao, K. and Schreer, G., 'Pets and Happiness: Examining the Association between Pet Ownership and Wellbeing', *Anthrozoös*, 29:2 (2016), pp. 283–96; Ambrose, G. *et al*, 'Is gardening associated with greater happiness of urban residents? A multi-activity, dynamic assessment in the Twin-Cities region, USA', *Landscape and Urban Planning*, June 2020.

p. 259 'Happiness can't be *pursued* …': Frankl, V., *Man's Search for Meaning* (Ebury, 2004).

INDEX

Note: italic page numbers indicate illustrations; the suffix 'n' a footnote on that page.

A

ability and disability, original meanings 241

abusive relationships, addiction to 214–15

academic performance and CNS stimulants 244

ACE (adverse childhood experiences) study 110–11

acronyms, disrespectful 27

addiction
beyond psychoactive substances 214; cocaine 185, 209, 212; combatting 216; definition 213; emergency medicine and 211–12; models of 214; schools of thought on 210–11; self-harming as 218–19; *see also* alcohol dependency

addictiveness of drugs aiding sleep 101, 107

ADHD (Attention-Deficit/Hyperactivity Disorder) 34, 61, 81n
ADDitude magazine 243; adult referrals 242; case history (Oscar) 236, 246; as diversity rather than disorder 242–3, 245–6; first description 241; low

mood and 119, 226; Procrastination Station support group 246; suspected case 226; treatment 243; use of CNS stimulants in 39, 119, 226, 236, 243–5

adrenaline
effects in anxiety 107; effects in bipolar illness 140; effects in panic 96, 97; and PTSD 132

Adventures in Human Being, by the author 218n

Aesculapius 37

Afghanistan 91, 127

Agata (patient with panic attacks) 104–5

agoraphobia 103

alcohol and pregnancy 222–4, 228
foetal alcohol syndrome 223–4, 228, 231, 246

alcohol dependency
case histories (Laura and Pauline) 206–8, 222–4; levels of consumption 209

Alcoholics Anonymous 215

Alzheimer, Alois 188, 190

American Center for Disease Control and Prevention (ACDC), on ADHD 242

childhood experiences
  abusive experiences as common 110–11; lasting influence 25, 61, 63–4; and mental distress 70; and substance addictions 214
childhood neglect 63–4
childhood sexual abuse 70–1, 80, 109–10, 117
children, naturalness of hope 258
children's secure unit 79–80, 81
children's stunted growth 245
chimpanzees 154, 191
Chinese Classification of Mental Disorders 28, 161
chlorpromazine, (Largactil) 99, 164, 192
choroid plexus 21
Churchill, Winston 162
'circular insanity,' bipolar illness as 144. 189
cirrhosis 209
city living and anxiety 89
Claire (newborn) 66–7
Clare, Tim 106
Cleomenes 181
cocaine addiction 185, 209, 212, 290
Coleridge, Samuel Taylor 147, 249
The Collected Schizophrenias, by Esmé Weijun Wang 179
communities, supportive 169, 173, 215–16, 218, 246
complex PTSD (cPTSD) 70, 114, 119–20
computer-games addiction 214, 223
concentration and ADHD 61, 243
connections, neural, in the brain 58
Connolly, John 44
consciousness
  emergence of 19–20, 22; flow of 57–8, 62–3, 84; Henry and William James on 57; nature of

2, 38, 57, 62; site of 74; whether perhaps ubiquitous 61
constellations of stars, impermanence *32*, 51
constellations of symptoms 31–3, 48, 51, 230
consultants, specialist psychiatrists as 24
consultations
  balance with the waiting room 122; Dr M's model 75–6; importance of listening 159–60, 252–3; psychiatric notes 148–9; specialist psychiatrists frameworks for 49
continuity of care 259
coping strategies
  addictions as 88; adopted in childhood 59, 80; psychosis as 99, 203; self-harm as 219–20; self-spells as 97; for those with autism 232; treatment focussed on 253
Cornelia de Lange syndrome 228
cost-effectiveness, children's support units 80
COVID-19 126
cranial nerves 17–19
Crichton, Alexander 241–2
crime, sanity and culpability 46, 116, 222
Crook, John 57
Csikszentmihalyi, Mihaly 257
Cuba, classification of mental disorders 28
cultural attitudes
  to constellations 51; and languages 126–7, 161; to mental illness 30, 32, 45–6, 50–1, 161, 193
cultural norms and society 46

Index

religion
   alternatives to medical help 162,
      216; and dissociation, after
      trauma 125; protecting against
      low mood 169, 254; and
      reverence for life 155
religious illumination and mania
      150
reward centres 210
rhythms of life 131, 152–3
Richard (patient with delusions)
      184–5
risk, categories of 43, 203
Robert (patient with learning
      disabilities) 228, 231, 246
Rogers, Carl 32
the Rosenhan experiment 46–7

S
Sacks, Oliver 41n, 221–2
safety, public, as purpose of
      detention 182–3
the Samaritans 175
Sanity, Madness and the Family, by
      Ronald Laing and Aaron
      Esterson 200–1
Sartre, Jean-Paul 29
Sauvages de Lacroix, François
      Boissier de 42
Saxena, Shekhar 30
schizoaffective disorder 27, 179
schizophrenia
   case histories (Helena, Brian,
      Erica and Cathy) 196–8, 202–4;
      coinage 189–90; different
      outcomes 199; first-rank
      symptoms 182, 204; hearing
      voices in 179; *The Initial
      Prodrome in Schizophrenia* 178;
      Insel on 57; mistaken diagnoses

   of 47–8, 200–1; risks in genetic
      groups 195; in twins 59
Schneider, Kurt 115, 182
Schou, Mogens 146
Scotland
   Outer Hebrides alcoholics 209;
      shock therapies 192
seasonal affective disorder (SAD)
      161, 167, 169
sedatives 107, 140
self-harm
   overlap with eating disorders
      218; sex differences 219–20
self-medication
   with alcohol or drugs 99, 148,
      208, 214, 216, 237; self-harm as
      219
self-preoccupation 100
self-spells 97
self-stimulation, electrical 210
semen loss anxiety 90
serotonin 39, 53–4, 60, 99, 167
sertraline 106, 139
sex addiction 61, 214, 220–1
Sexual Psychopathology, by Krafft-
      Ebing 45
Shapeshifters, by the author 217n
Shawn, Allen 100
Sherrington, Charles 63–4
'shit-life syndrome' 27, 159, 167
shock therapies 192–3
side-effects
   of amphetamines 119, 245; of
      anticonvulsants 208; of
      antidepressants 169; of
      antipsychotics 203; of lithium
      145, 146; of tranquillisers 164
Silberman, Steve 246
Singer, Judy 230
slavery 202
sleep